Just a Word

Rose Lamatt

Just a Word: Friends encounter Alzheimer's
by Rose Lamatt. Copyright © 2009

For information, www.rmlamatt.com

ISBN: 1-1440475172
ISBN: 13-9781440475177

Just a Word
Friends encounter Alzheimer's

Rose Lamatt

Also by Rose Lamatt

Don't Look Forward

For Carol, and other victims of Alzheimer's, and for Rose, and other caregivers.

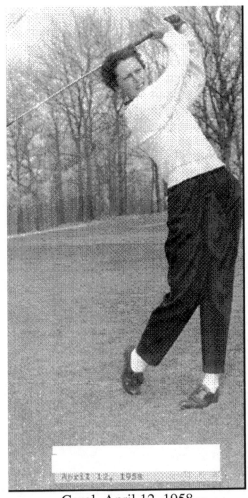

Carol, April 12, 1958

Prologue

On a Tuesday morning in November 1985, I drank a cup of coffee with my husband, then walked with him to the door and said goodbye. I watched him walk down the brick walkway, his gait fast, then climb into his company car. 'Be gone all day and night,' he had said.

I had known him all my life. He was my brother's best friend, and had shared meals with us. Growing up I played stickball, tag and other games with him and the kids on the block. At twenty he was in the Navy—tall and in his sailor whites, stood out in a crowd. How excited I was when he bought his first car, a red and white convertible. At home on leave he picked me up at school with the top down, and I jumped in giving him a peck on the cheek. He put his arm around me and we drove away, me waving to my girlfriends. The next day they told me how lucky I was, what a great 'catch' he was. Every seventeen-year-old girl's dream—a convertible and a good-looking sailor. I had it all.

I heard our daughter running water in the upstairs bathroom, probably bushing her teeth, getting ready for school. Our twenty-year-old son lay in bed after a night on the town with friends. It was the perfect American family: husband, wife, two children, dog, cat, a large colonial house with three cars, a country club membership, and everything money could buy. At forty, I was living the life I had dreamed.

Working on another cup of coffee, I waited for my daughter to come down stairs. Thoughts of the priest's words in 1962 came, 'Til death do you part'. Twenty-one years married. Where did they go? Why did they change?

After seeing my daughter on the bus, I waved and whispered, "*Goodbye Hope.*" I wiped a tear, turned and walked back to the house. Looking at it, I thought how beautiful the big colonial still was. I remembered our Sunday drives before marriage, looking at large houses in up scaled neighborhoods on the north shore of Long Island. "I want one like that," I had said. And he answered, 'Sure, okay.' Seemed ages ago. *It was.*

Looking at the brass knocker, I grinned. You always wanted one of those, didn't you? But no one ever used it. Maybe around Christmas or Halloween—other than that, it never sounded. I pulled back the knocker for old time sake, letting it mash against the plate.

Closing the door, the corner of my eye caught a glimpse of the black baby grand piano, by the windows. Going to it, I rolled back the top and pressed middle C, *pure sound.* The instrument and my painting had kept me sane when agoraphobia smothered me, afraid to go out, even to the mailbox at the end of the driveway. I'd stay in all day until one of the kids came home from school, to fill the void. I'd wait for Ed to food shop. I waited on him for everything.

Now at the 'black beauty', I played Chopin Etudes, and tears came. Played notes the way the composer had meant them, heart-breaking sounds. He was my favorite, and always would be. I looked out the window at the pines we had planted. How tall they'd gotten. (I had lost inches due to scoliosis worsening.) I looked at the cherry wood writers' desk, where I had spent little time. I loved its look, especially the forest green leather chair that kept it company. I gazed around the room, remembering how I danced alone when we moved in. I'd blast the stereo speakers: Puccini, Sinatra or Mathis flowing from them, making me *feel*.

I got up, climbed the wood staircase admiring its shine. My steps echoed through the house. At the top, I turned toward the closed door. What time had *he* come in last night, or was it early morning? Did he drink so much that he couldn't drive? His car wasn't in the driveway when I said goodbye to Ed. Had he drank like his father, and my father? I hoped not, but in my heart, I expected so. He was fun to raise until age seventeen. Before that he'd been my little friend, during panic attacks and agoraphobia. I'd converse with him of God, conversations most mothers and sons didn't have. I felt our relationship a gift. Now, twenty, he was different. He thought he knew it all, and there wasn't any more I could teach him.

My daughter was different; she *did* know it all at thirteen, a smart child at two, old mentally for her age. She was a good child, and had a mind of her own. I didn't have to teach her anything. I tried at times, but she didn't listen, and did things her way. She was thirteen going on thirty, but that was okay.

I climbed the stairs to the attic getting two suitcases. I packed clothes I'd need, then showered and dressed in jeans, a shirt, and sneakers. I took my gray jacket out of the closet. I'd take just enough, nothing more. I would leave the rest to *him* and the kids. He could have the material things. I wanted a different life, away from drinking. I wanted a new life.

Before descending the stairs, I looked toward the closed door, '*Goodbye Matthew*'.

Downstairs I waited for the car—the car that would take me somewhere else. I saw it come up the driveway and felt warm inside. Warmth that told me I was following my Journey. The horn blew short. I closed the door behind me and walked down the brick walkway, covering Ed's footprints.

1

C arol, dinner's ready," I called from the kitchen.

We had taken showers and changed into shorts after a hot day of golf. I fixed a meal of leftovers, ham, potatoes and cabbage while Carol read the newspaper on the screened porch. Walking toward her, I see how tan she is, her long legs the color of bronze.

I first spotted those long legs ten years ago, coming up the eighteenth fairway at a country club on Long Island. She walked almost to background music, her feet gliding atop the grass, not touching ground. She was tall, I could see—much taller than me. She walked with another by her side, pulling golf carts. I stood at the side entrance to the clubhouse, unable to move or think. She held my gaze. I had never seen anyone so perfect to the eye, and thought I knew her. I asked the person I was playing with who she was? Joeie, my friend told me her name was Carol Beinbrink, one of the best golfers on Long Island, and I remembered then reading about her years ago in local newspapers. *The next Babe Zaharias.*

That's all I knew of Carol that day, but as time went on, I met her at a tournament she was running for cancer. When

I did get a chance to play with her a few years later, I found her to be a great competitor, courteous, compassionate, loving and giving, and felt lucky to have met her. Everyone at the club loved her, and I could not imagine why she would befriend a fearful fool like me.

My life before her had been one of fear: fear of dying, fear of being alone, fear of people, fear of going out, fear, fear, fear, all since the age of sixteen. I had never really been happy. My prayers each night for two years were, *Please send me someone to make me happy.*

I'm convinced God answered my prayers. Sometimes we meet people we think we've met before, we know them as if they've been out best friend, somewhere, sometime. I don't have answers. I only know what I felt that day I first saw Carol.

In the coming years, I became closer to her than I'd ever been to anyone before. I looked up to her for everything. She taught me to laugh and be a kid again, the kid who loved life, riding a bike, sledding down a hill in winter, the kid who saw the good in everything and everyone. I'd lost that kid at sixteen, when I became afraid to live.

That day I walked away from the big beautiful colonial, and climbed into her waiting car in the driveway, was the start of my new life. We came to Jupiter, Florida where I enjoyed the life God had planned for me. We played in golf leagues from Fort Pierce to Fort Lauderdale, loving every minute, making a pact to smile at everyone we met, and thanking God each morning we had two feet on the floor. We were happy serving others. My life had done a three hundred and sixty degree turn, from someone who feared everything, hated living and wanted life to end, to someone who couldn't get enough of life. God had blessed me with this person named Carol.

Now, five years later calling her to dinner she looks exactly like the oil portrait hanging over our couch, taken in her twenties, some forty years ago. *She hasn't changed at all.* I've started graying around the face, producing a halo affect and wear glasses. She's sixteen years older than I, and looks fantastic.

"What are you reading?" I ask, stepping onto the porch.

"A story about a woman named The Pelican Lady. She saves pelicans that have swallowed fishhooks or have broken wings. Look Rose, she keeps them in cages until they're able to fly, then lets them go."

I looked at the picture and article, saying how lucky we were to be living here.

"Yep, you're right about that. Jupiter was always my little spot of heaven."

"Dinner's ready, we really should eat before it gets late. What do you want to drink?"

Water, she says, and I take two glasses from the kitchen cabinet, filling them with ice water, throwing in a slice of lemon. With our nightly prayer said, we eat and talk of the day's golf. We had played in Boca.

"What did you get on the ninth hole?" I ask.

"I pared it, but it was a tuff little par three. It sure had a lot of trouble around it."

"You're telling me. I wound up with a six. I couldn't believe it, six, on a par three. The water in front of the green was deceiving. I hit on the upslope to the green, and it rolled all the way back into the drink."

She tells me of her opponent, "She out drove me every hole. I don't think I saw anyone hit such a long ball."

"Really? Where was she from?"

"Stuart, I think."

"Gee, we should have asked her to drive down with us."

I tell her about the gal I played against, one putting twelve greens, and beating me.

Nearing the end of dinner, Carol's eyes fix on the ceiling, and she begins shaking her head.

"Ca?"

No answer, still shaking.

"Ca, are you okay?"

Nothing.

I grab her shoulders, "*Ca— CAROL!*" She stops and looks at me.

"Are you all right?"

"Yes, why?" snapping out of it.

"Are you sure you're okay?"

"Yes, I'm fine. Why, what's the matter?"

"You were shaking your head, staring at the ceiling. You sure you feel all right?"

"Yes. I guess I didn't hear you."

"Ca, you were somewhere else. Do you have any pain?"

"No, I'm fine. I didn't drink enough water today, maybe that's it. I was thirsty all day."

"You need to stop drinking soda and drink more water. Would you please do that, *for me*?"

"I'll try...okay, let's forget it."

Something happened. I know. But she seems okay now. I pour decaf coffee, and get four chocolate chip cookies, two a piece, but I can't let go of what I saw. I'd never seen anything like it before.

Weeks later, playing golf, Carol doesn't remember where she's hit the ball. It's slightly off the fairway when I show her. She's always been down the middle since our first game in 1983.

Soon I'm beating her, when in all the years I never have. Her swing is shorter, but she still out drives me.

Head tremors are more, and I convince her to see Dr. Ban our doctor since we moved to Jupiter. The nurse checks her blood pressure and pulse, "Seems fine," she says. The doctor comes in, and shakes our hands.

"Hello, how are you two doing? Still beating all those golfers in Palm Beach?"

"No, not really. Carol's having difficulty," I answer.

He turns to Carol. "What's happening with you?"

"Rose thought I should make an appointment. She's concerned something's wrong."

"Oh…and what's that?" looking at Carol, then me.

"She says my head shakes and I stare at the ceiling. She says I forget where I've hit the golf ball."

Seated, I observe, making sure she tells him everything. He turns to me. I tell him what I've seen, pretty much the same as she's told him.

"Let me check your lungs and listen to your heart." I watch. "Okay, now your reflexes." Her foot jumps as he hits her knee with the rubber hammer. "Watch my finger," he says. Her eyes move back and forth, then up and down, after his finger. "Lay down," he presses on her stomach, checks her armpits and ankles. "Let's get some blood work just to make sure everything's okay. It's probably your heart medication. Sometimes medications can make the brain do strange things. In fact, let's change it to something else." Pulling a script pad from his pocket, he writes a new prescription. We shake hands and say goodbye, he sends in the nurse.

"Oh boy, I hate this," my friend says.

"It'll only take a minute," says the nurse. But after the third try, Carol's making faces. I watch, feeling for her, knowing she's in pain. The nurse repeats, "I'm sorry, you have rollover veins. I guess they're tired and want to go to sleep." This gets a smile from Carol. Finally, the needle hits home and I watch her blood flow into tubes while she looks the other way.

On the way home, we stop to fill the new prescription and get ice cream. After all she's been through she deserves it.

Two days later the nurse calls, saying, blood work's normal, and the doctor wants her to take the new medication for her mitral valve prolapse. Days later she's worse. Standing, she's dizzy, has heart palpitations and feels she's going to pass out. Soon she doesn't want to leave the house and I fully understand why.

Another medication is tried. "We have to find the right one that will stop your palpitations," says the doctor. And orders more blood work and extensive testing— neurological tests, cardiac tests, an MRI of the brain. A month we go from doctor to doctor, test after test.

An EEG without sleep, she stays awake twenty-four hours. I want to be with her and do, until two in the morning, when I go to bed. At four-thirty, using the bathroom, I see her watching television.

"See, I'm not sleeping," she says. "I'm wide awake," and smiles.

"Would you like a cup of tea? I'll keep you company."

"You don't have to. Go back to bed. I won't go to sleep."

"I know you won't, but I'd like to be with you." Like the picture she gave years ago for Christmas. Albert Camus words, 'Don't walk in front of me I may not follow. Don't walk behind me I may not lead. Just walk beside me and be my friend'. I make tea and we play gin rummy. At six I make pancakes and eggs. By eight-thirty, we're at the doctor's office for another test. Normal. All tests are normal, but her head tremors continue.

The final test, a spinal tap, is checking for encephalitis. The neurologist comes in where we've been waiting for two hours, telling us, he's sorry he's late. He had an emergency. He tells Carol to lie on her side and pull her knees up to her chest. "This will only take a few minutes," he says. I see the long needle come out of his bag and head to the hallway. When finished he meets me there.

"What do you think is wrong?" I ask.

"I don't know. If this comes back normal, then I would suggest a PET scan."

"What happens if the test shows positive?"

"Then she'll be treated."

"I hope it shows something."

"I need to go. I'm late for another patient. I'll call you when the results are in. Figure a few days."

"Thanks, Doc."

The doctor's office calls saying the test is normal, and within a week we are headed to Long Island for a PET scan. Carol's gotten the name of a doctor from a golf friend, and has made an appointment. We take the train, because I don't feel confident driving the distance. The train is full, people going north for Thanksgiving. We play gin rummy to pass time, and eat in the dining car to be around people. Carol meets a man she played golf with years ago in Pinehurst, North Carolina and the twenty-one hour trip to Grand Central Station goes faster.

Once on Long Island, the receptionist shows us to a waiting room. I'm at a loss for words, not knowing what to expect. I see Carol's worried look, me thinking, am I seeing my reflection on her face? The nurse calls Carol's name. Dr. Greenberg is good-looking, young, with glasses and black hair. He has that smart look about him, top-of-class smart—just a feeling.

"So what brings you to me?"

"My friend, Judith Packerson, recommended you. Here, I brought my records from Florida," Carol hands him the bulging folder.

"So you know Judy?" as he takes the overstuffed folder. "She's a great golfer." And settles back in his chair, studying papers. I watch his fingers turn pages, months of testing.

"This is good. Looks like you've had everything done."

Ca, smiles, "Yes, you could say that."

"We won't repeat any tests. Right now, I'd like to ask you some questions."

"Do you want me to leave?" I ask. He says I can stay.

"Carol, I'm going to give you three words to remember. Then I'll ask you to repeat them later. The words are: boat, pencil, TV."

"Boat, pencil, TV," she repeats.

"What day is it?"

"Friday."

"What month is it?"

"November."

"Who is the president?"

"President Reagan," she answers.

"What season is it?"

"Fall."

"Starting with one hundred, subtract seven from the last number."

"93...86...79..."

I sit amazed, as she subtracts seven from every number while I count on the fingers in my lap, thinking, *if I were taking the test I'd fail.*

"Very good," he stops her, gives her a blank sheet of paper. "Draw the face of a clock with the hands on two-thirty."

I watch, stupid. She knows how to tell time. Why aren't you doing some other test?

I look at the clock she's drawn. It's small, but the hands read two-thirty.

"Can you tell me the three words I asked you to remember?" he asks.

She puts her finger to her lips, and closes her eyes.

"TV, boat, and uh…car."

Something's different. I remember two words, *TV* and *boat* but don't think the third was *car*.

"You did fine. Now we'll go down the hall for a PET scan. Rose, have a seat here," and opens the door for Carol.

"Okay, see you later, Ca."

"Yep, see you later," she says smiling.

I sit outside the room, and pick up a magazine. *The doctor said, about forty-five minutes.* I look at pictures, not reading words attached. I wonder what she's going through. *Is she seriously ill? Why haven't they found anything? What more is there to look for?*

Maybe there's *nothing* wrong. I'm so tired of doctors and tests. First me, with heart problems, now her with God knows what?

The technician comes out, "You can go in now—we're finished."

I see Carol tying her sneakers. "Thank God that's over."

The technician tells us the doctor wants to see both of us in his office.

She looks so healthy. How can there be anything wrong with her? I think, walking down the hall. She tells me of loud noises she heard while in the tube.

Dr. Greenberg sits in his office, "You did fine, Carol," then says he needs to read the scan and will let us know Monday morning. I give him the motel phone number.

Today is Friday. More days of waiting. We shake hands, thanking him, and are out the door into a cold wind that has picked up since we arrived three hours ago. The weather report said possible frost tonight.

Once off the Long Island Expressway, I tell her we need chocalotta ice cream. She agrees, "Make mine a hot fudge sundae."

"You're entitled after all you've been through. I don't know how you stood it, in that tube. Talk about claustrophobia."

I remember the days we went for chocolate ice cream sodas after a hot day of golf on Long Island and she'd say, 'I think we need some *chocalotta* ice cream,' I thought the name neat, and kept it.

Back at the motel Mom has left a message to call her. I return the call, and she asks, "How'd it go today?"

I tell her it went well, but we don't know anything yet. "Come for dinner," she says. "Paul and Donna are going to be here."

"What are you making?" I ask loud enough so Carol can hear, in case she doesn't want to go. However, she nods, 'yes'.

Mom says she's made sauce with meatballs and sausage, asking if I want linguini or spaghetti. I say spaghetti, and we'll bring desert.

"No, don't bring dessert. The freezer is full of pie and cake."

I hear John in the background, "Tell her to bring cheese strudel."

"Hush, John," Mom says. "Be quiet."

"No, tell her to bring strudel," John yells louder.

I remember when my mother didn't have a say in the household I grew up in with my father. I'm sorry Dad has passed on, but glad Mom is happy with John. He makes her laugh, and I miss them both, since I moved to Florida, but this is life. It changes, hopefully for the best, and for Mom it has.

"Mom, I hear him. I'll pick up strudel. If you need help, let me know. We'll be here for the rest of the afternoon. We left at six this morning and we're very tired."

"Tell Carol we said hello."

"I will—see you later," and set the phone down.

We lay down for a nap and Carol is snoring within minutes. I, on the other hand, think of the morning's adventure and have too many questions.

Dinner was just what we needed. John played the piano and sung while Mom ran around making sure everyone had enough to eat and drink. She loved seeing people enjoy themselves. The spaghetti and meatballs were just as I remembered as a child. Growing up I knew she was a *good* Italian cook, and had taught me everything I knew. But, I didn't have that special something, a touch of this and a touch of that—no measuring cups with her.

Doing dishes later, with my sister-in-law Donna, she asks, "When will you have the results of Carols test?"

"The doctor said probably Monday."

"How's she doing? She looks nervous."

"I guess she is a little nervous. I'm nervous not knowing what's wrong. But, you know her, she takes one step at a time." I hear her in the living room laughing with John and talking golf with my brother. When Donna and I join the group, Mom brings out an old photo album. I see pictures of Ed, and the kids, along with pictures of me as a child with my parents and brothers.

Pointing to one of Paul, it shows how much hair he used to have. He's just about bald now, having the look of a Monk. "Hey, Ca, look how much hair Paul used to have," making fun of him. "Look how wavy and dark it used to be."

"Paul jumps right back at me, "You wait and see you're going to lose yours some day."

At that, I run my hands through my dark thick hair carrying the gray halo. "Oh no, I'm not."

Everyone laughs while brother and sister discuss their heads, and I miss that banter we used to have. I've forgotten how much my brothers meant to me when I was young. With both my parents working I was home alone most of the time, and if it wasn't for their guiding hands that kept me in line, God know what trouble I'd be in.

At ten o'clock, we said goodnight, leaving behind a stressful day, followed by an evening filled with love. Mom had looked happy, but I knew she, too, worried about Carol.

Saturday, we played golf and had lunch at the club, and I remember the Ladies Club championships with Joeie and Carol. Sunday we picked up Hope for church, and met Mom while John sang in the choir upstairs. Just like old times, together filling one pew. Ed and Matthew, were the only ones missing. Prayers went up for Carol, and a 'thank you' for Mom still here. She'd had a few rough years; cancer of the breast, and a heart attack. I'm glad she's still around. Dad had passed away right after Ed and I adopted Hope.

After church, having breakfast at the town diner, Hope asks, "When are you going back to Florida?"

"Next week I suppose. It's getting too cold." and see Mom's face drop at my words. I know she hates it every year when I say, 'it's time to go back to Florida'. I miss her and know she misses me. We had spent a lot of time together after I got married, more than before. Funny, I remember her saying just before I got married. 'Well, I guess I won't see you much after you're married.' And I had told her, 'don't be crazy, I'll see you more. We'll go shopping all the time.' And that's just what we did, especially after I quit work and got pregnant. We went shopping, at least three times a week and had lunch afterwards, enjoying each others company. More than when I was young. Mom was always there for me, always willing to baby sit when Ed and I went out. She lived with us for a short period, and I loved having her in my days of fear, even though she didn't know I was afraid of dying at the time. She was a comfort to me, but I never told her why. I think she knew without me telling her. Why don't we tell people we love how much they mean to us, at the time?

Now she changes the subject of leaving and asks, "Will we see you tomorrow?"

I tell her yes, but we have to wait for the doctor's phone call first. "Maybe we can get together in the afternoon for lunch and shopping."

Hope jumps in giving us a rundown of classes, and what's happening in the boyfriend department. She says she'll be down to visit us during winter recess.

The new school she's attending seems to be working out. She's meeting kids from all over the world, and I'm glad she's not the only Oriental in her class, as she used to be. She's looking forward to college. *I'm glad.*

2

Monday morning I run down to the motel's continental breakfast, bringing back cereal, bananas, and coffee. Just finishing coffee, the phone rings. I look at Carol, then pick up the receiver.

"Hello?"

"Good morning. How are you this morning?" Dr. Greenberg asks.

"Fine, thank you." I'd been waiting for this call. We both had been waiting, but not mentioned in words. I'm sure it's nothing, maybe a gland problem they haven't found yet, or a blood disorder not picked up. In New York, we had the best doctor's and hospitals. I was sure someone would find what was wrong with her, and finally asked, "Do you have any news for us?"

He goes into a long explanation of Carol's PET scan and the other test. Some I understand, most I don't.

"I'm sorry to tell you Rose, Carol has a dementia disease known as Alzheimer's."

I heard him, yet not. I ask him to repeat it. Again, I hear the word, *Alzheimer's.* I stand from my safe sitting spot on the bed. I can't say anything and want him to take back the 'word'.

I'm unable to say anything while he finishes telling me his findings. "Thank you," I say and hang up.

Thank you? Thank you for what? You don't thank someone for this *word*. You thank someone when they say God bless you, after you sneeze, or when they give you a gift. This wasn't a sneeze or a gift. There wasn't anything to say Thank you for?

Carol, reading by the window, looks at me.

"Who was it?"

I can't answer.

"Was it the doctor?"

I hear, but don't know what to say. I need to get my thoughts in order.

Alzheimer's? How? Why? Where did she get it? How bad is it?

Again, as in a distance she asks, "What is it?"

"Oh, it's nothing." How do I tell her when I don't believe it. How do I do this? There were no lessons in school on this. How do you tell someone they're ill, or possibly going to die? Who knows what will happen? We never used this word. We didn't know anyone who had this word. After a few minutes I put *my* words together, "Yes, that was the doctor."

"Well, what did he say?"

I look at her, feeling pity—no, sorrow—no, nothing. I'm numb, in shock. Like a robot, I speak, "The doctor says you have Alzheimer's disease."

She stares at me for what seems a long time. Then her eyes go wide, and then she closes them. Her mouth forms an O as she throws back her head, '*Oh, my God...No!*' Her hands cover her face and she leans forward, her body shakes with hard sobs. I go to her, kneel on the floor and hold her.

"Oh God," she cries. And my heart cries along with her. "I'll need to go into a nursing home," she says.

"No—no, you won't. We'll go through this together. I promise. Maybe they're wrong, maybe they made a mistake." I cry with her, letting her know we *will* go through this together.

Somewhere tucked in my heart, I know the love between us is stronger than any illness. That alone will cure her. *I know YOU will hear our cries, dear Lord.*

In bed I pull the cover up around us, and hold her for a long time. The phone rings. I pick it up.

"Hello, Rose? I just got off the phone with Dr. Greenberg. I'm sorry to hear about Carol. If there's anything I can do, please call me." Dr. Ban from Florida.

I thank him for calling and say we'll be home in a few days, no more comes out of me.

I decide to call Mom, telling her I have one of my migraines, and we'll see her tomorrow. I don't mention the word Alzheimer's. For the rest of the day we stay in our room, sending out for dinner. The day is lost, like us.

The next two days I tell family and some friends the news. For them, like us, it's hard to believe and soon we're headed south on a train. We stay in our compartment playing gin rummy or staring out a window, not believing the new word Alzheimer's.

3

When home, friends and neighbors are just as surprised as we are, but I find, if we live without the word our days are almost normal.

As Christmas approaches, we go all-out, decorating. It's been an awful year, my heart condition detected, caused by a flu I had when I was sixteen, and then Alzheimer's. It's been a nightmare, and we've forgotten *how* to laugh. We deserve a happy Christmas.

Carol retrieves ornaments from storage while I move furniture, making space for the tree. We sing carols, tossing tinsel on the tree like kids. Neighbors come with fruitcakes and candy canes, and phone calls come from the north. The dining table decorated with sprigs of pine and pinecones, and a large glass bowl sits in the center, holding colored Christmas balls. Carol shines silverware and brass candlestick holders, filling them with red candles. A wreath made of fruit hangs on the door, and a new teddy bear wearing a red Santa hat and scarf sits in a chair playing Christmas carols.

For dinner, I make cornish hens stuffed with apple, cooked with peaches and prunes, green beans, salad, fresh rolls, and chocolate cake for dessert. One neighbor joins us with her new knee replacement and another who has no one. The evening is meaningful, shared with friends. Later, we ready ourselves for our traditional Christmas Eve mass. We're tired this year, not as energetic as other years, but we make the evening complete by out singing everyone in church. From my heart and soul, I pray all illness be gone.

Neither of us know much about this new disease that has attacked our little family. All we know is it's bad, so in the coming weeks we talk to the Alzheimer's Association. We're told a support group meets once a week, close by, and Carol insists on going. At our first meeting, we see two faces we recognize, Linda and Ray. The couple that decorated our condo in '86. Ray is facilitator of the group, his brother has Alzheimer's. It's good to see old friends, to know we have something in common besides drapes and couches. The group is small, maybe ten or twelve people, all caregivers. Melinda, a nurse, is visiting guest speaker, and greets everyone.

We listen how everyone's week went. Some folks ran out of houses in nightgowns, in the middle of the night, while caregivers called police to find them. One woman, Leone, talks of her father breaking water pipes, thinking he's still a plumber. Horror stories, I want to leave. We don't belong here. These folks are different from us. *Why did we come?*

Melinda makes her way to us, and asks names.

"My name is Carol. I have Alzheimer's."

My God, I didn't think she was going to blurt it out like that. I knew her to be open but not this open. Yet, somewhere deep inside myself I'm proud of her.

"Good to have you with us, Carol."

Next, all eyes are on me. "My name is Rose and I live with Carol." *There, that wasn't so bad.*

Melinda smiles saying, "Welcome to the group, girls. You'll find we have a lot of fun here. How can we help you?"

"I want to know if there's a cure?" asks Carol.

"No, not yet, but they're working on it. There's a research center in Tamarac doing studies. I'll have the Alzheimer's Association call you with the number."

"Thank you," answers Carol.

Me next, "What age does a person get this disease? Could a person have a wrong diagnosis?" From what I've deducted, Carol is the youngest in the group, diagnosed at age sixty-four.

"It was once considered a young person's disease— as early as thirty—but they're finding more elderly people with it now. It used to be called senility." Everyone nods. "As far as a true diagnosis, the only one I know of is a brain biopsy, after death."

After death? I think, and thank Melinda.

We listen to unbelievable stories and I remember an old woman who lived across the street from us when I was growing up. Me and other kids played stickball on the street, and would see her taken away in a black car. She'd stare back at us through the window, and we thought she was crazy, taken away by the paddy wagon, we called it. Her son eventually put her in an institution. *Could this be the same disease?*

On the way home, no words are said, in mind, I'm still at the meeting. At dinner I tell her, "I don't think we should go to those meetings again. You're not sick, and besides, we're busy everyday, playing golf, riding our bikes, swimming, and walking the heart trail. You're not like them."

Carol agrees.

On February 14th she turns sixty-five, looking more like forty-five. She has a full head of hair, no gray, the picture of health. At her request, I make shrimp and spaghetti, chocolate cake and add sixty-five candles, just for fun. Friends and neighbors join us for the big blow out as she laughs, happy.

A phone call comes from the Alzheimer's Association asking if she wants to join an adult Day Care Center. "She doesn't need day care," I say. "We're doing just fine. I don't even think she has the disease." There, I told them.

4

As the months pass, Carol's tremors increase. She leaves clothing or paper work out of place scattered around the house. She'd been neat, organized, teaching me to be. Now she looks for something, not knowing where she's left it. She drives wherever we go and I worry. At dinner, I bring the subject up, saying we should discuss her driving.

"Yes, what about it?" she says.

Hard to find the right words, I tell her if she's in an accident and its known she has Alzheimer's, she will be held responsible.

"You want me to quit driving?"

"Well … no, not really." I don't have the heart to say 'yes'. "Maybe you should ask your advisor, okay?"

She agrees and speaks with her advisor who recommends she stop driving. *'I'm right. I hate it.'*

I call the research center, make an appointment, she'll get on a drug that will stop this disease.

Carol writes in her little black daily entry book: 7:30 a.m. Dr. Mike, Neuro Med Center for Res.

Anticipating the trip the night before, I'm unable to sleep. If you wanted to know about Alzheimer's, this was the place to go. But, I don't think she has it. I'm sure it's something they haven't found a name for yet.

The drive south is long, due to commuter traffic. "We'll make a day of it," I tell her. "Go shopping, and have a nice lunch out." She likes the idea.

With me driving, and Carol the map-reader, we find the center easily. The waiting room is small, ten or so chairs. A glass window slides back, "Hi, first time here?" the receptionist asks.

"Yes"—come two voices in unison.

"Please fill these out," she says, handing us at least ten sheets of paper. "I'm sorry there's a wait. We're backed up a little, so have a seat and make yourselves comfortable."

Papers on both laps, we start with the first page. Carol writes her name, address, social security and insurance numbers, I watch. Next, your doctor, and history, I help. All records are with us; lab work, Dr. Ban's reports, Dr. Greenberg's, everything she's gone through for months. I deliver the filled pages to the woman behind the glass, and we sit and wait. I pick up a magazine I used to read with my children while waiting in doctor's offices. A fun magazine, pages of pictures where you have to find the hidden hammer, pineapple, or other items on the page. It keeps us busy.

An hour later, we hear Carol's name called. We're led down a long hallway, doors jutting off it. We enter a room, and sit in front of a large mahogany desk.

"Dr. Mike will be in shortly," the nurse says.

I look out the window, Carol's eyes follow.

A young man, maybe in his late thirties, early forties, comes in. "Hello, I'm Dr. Mike."

I stand and say, "Nice to meet you. I'm Rose," then motion to my friend, "This is Carol."

"Hello," she says, and reaches her hand out, as she did with me when we met for club championships.

The doctor has a friendly, relaxed manner. Sitting, he opens the folder the nurse has left on his desk. "How was the drive?"

"The traffic was heavy, but not bad," I answer.

"So you're in Jupiter?" he asks. "Are you there year round?"

"Yes, except when we go north to visit family on Long Island."

"I like Jupiter. I take my wife and son fishing off the Inlet on weekends."

"No kidding? We live close to the Inlet. We moved there in '85." I see Carol playing with her fingernails, seemingly nervous, yet smiling.

Medical questions come, "Why do you want research? What led you here?" and more, as he thumbs through the stack of papers we have brought him.

Finished with questions and answers he tells me to wait in the outer room. I get up, and turn to Carol. "See you later, kiddo."

"See ya," she answers with that soft look she's had, since I met her.

I wait, thinking my new thoughts. Dr. Mike will help her, I know. She's not really sick. They'll find that out here. This is the place to be, I'm sure.

Forty-five minutes later Carol comes out with the nurse saying, "Rose, Dr. Mike wants to see you."

"Oh, okay." And return to the same room as before.

He greets me again saying, "Carol's gone down the hall for testing."

I nod.

"She's very nice, Rose, but she *is* confused at times."

"I think I'd be too, after all she's been through. So many months of doctors and tests, with no diagnosis, then up north where she's diagnosed with Alzheimer's. I'm sure she's in shock. I know I am."

Then I spill all the past months questions, and more. 'Where did it come from? How did she get it? Could it be something else?' On and on I go, happy venting.

Dr. Mike lets me, offering no answers.

"What's she like at home?"

"She's fine, except for her head shaking and leaving some things out of place. I really don't think she has Alzheimer's."

"I'm afraid the PET scan shows she has some form of dementia."

"But she's so organized! I do most of the cooking. She makes breakfast sometimes, but she's never cooked meals in all the time I've known her. We clean the house together and she handles all the bills and finances. How does someone do that, and have dementia?"

He looks at me almost as if wanting to say, 'I'm sorry,' but says instead, "She's in the very beginning stages. The disease can go from three to twenty-one years. We don't know very much about it."

I tell him: she plays golf, she rides her bike, she swims, we shop together, she reads books and the newspaper, watches the investments on TV, goes to the movies. How could she be sick?

He asks what foods she eats.

"We eat healthy, mostly fresh foods: fruits, vegetables, fish, chicken—all the right things you're supposed to do. We don't eat red meat or fatty foods, because of my heart problem. I was diagnosed with Ventricle Tachycardia in 1990."

"Does she smoke?"

"No. We both quit in '88 when I started having palpitations. You know something weird, though. We both had palpitations at the same time. Hers followed mine, and that's when they found she had mitral valve prolapse. I even wondered if it's something in the air, or our apartment, or the golf course. One day on the course we saw dead fish floating on the ponds."

"I don't know Rose. You know there's no medication for Alzheimer's."

"Yes, our doctor told us that. That's why we're here, hoping *you* can help."

"Well, after her blood work and testing is done, she'll be put on a drug of choice. It will be a double-blind study, which means you don't know if you're getting the drug or not."

"You mean she won't get the real drug?" I ask, surprised.

"We won't know if it's a placebo or the drug. The only people who know are the companies that make the drug."

"You mean *you* won't know either?"

"No, only the drug company. Then she'll be tested each month when you bring her. You *will* bring her?"

"Oh, yes. I'll bring her, we live together."

"She'll have blood work and take other tests that will be sent to the drug firm."

I understand, but then, don't. *How can the doctor not know if she's on the real drug?* I ask more questions, getting more tired each minute. God knows what Carol is feeling?

Dr. Mike's behind in appointments and leads me to where Carol's having blood work done. Poor Ca, she hates that, because of those rollover veins, but she hangs in there like a real trouper. Then, we're sent to the hospital behind the center.

"How'd the testing go, Ca?" I ask as we walk.

"Not bad, but some questions were really stupid. The woman asked me if I could tie my shoelaces."

Ummm, what do I say to that? "Well, I guess they're set questions for everyone, not just you." I don't want her to feel different.

We get exercise taking the stairs to the third floor where she's to have an EEG. I'm allowed to stay and watch my friend on a table. I wonder what she thinks as flashing white lights happen above her, while a machine spits paper on the floor. The paper shows rows of lines, straight and wavy, up then down. *All done before without lights. Do the lights make a difference?* Thank God she doesn't need to repeat the MRI.

We see Dr. Mike in his office at day's end and he tells us his plan of attack. "Carol qualifies for three studies," he says, handing us three manila envelopes. "Read the material carefully, and then pick the study you want."

We listen, hopeful. I know she'll be cured, if not through medicine, then through all our prayers.

I tell the receptionist we're staying at a motel on the beach tonight, can she make an early morning appointment, we sure would appreciate it.

"How about eight o'clock?"

"That's fine, thank you," I say.

I know Carol must be tired. I sure am. We stop for dinner, then wind up at the same motel I had been with Ed and the kids years ago, when we came to Florida. It's small. One that's quiet. After check in, that familiar look comes back. Funny, I'm at the same motel after so many years, under different circumstances. Not watching kids laugh in the pool now, or catch a wave with their father, this time it's sickness.

We retrieve two chairs from the car trunk and settle to watch waves. High tide is beautiful, blue-green water. Carol quickly falls asleep. I watch waves, and her. *She's so peaceful. Why is that other life out there...the worried one? I wish life could always be like this. It used to.*

Later in our room, we go over drug studies; two from Europe, one from the United States used for another illness, now being tested on the Alzheimer's brain.

I call Paul, my brother who is a pharmacist for his opinion. He knows the US drug and assures me it's safe. It has few side effects. We're confident it's the right choice.

The next morning, after breakfast, we return to the center, and tell Dr. Mike our choice. We sign papers as if our lives depend on it—in a sense, one does. He explains how the study works, office visits for blood work and Carol's given plain white boxes. We make our next appointment for later in the day, hoping to miss heavy traffic, and say goodbye. We leave with a feeling of hope, hidden inside boxes.

Starving, we stop for tuna sandwiches and lemonade. I see a look of happiness on her and feel it within myself. After lunch, we buy bagels for us, and neighbors.

Taking the long way home along Route 1, we drive through small towns, passing homes on Palm Beach Island. It's longer, but relaxing. Arriving home late afternoon, neighbors, Jay and Bea, are on the catwalk. "Welcome home," they say, as they do when we come back from our northern trips.

"Wait till you see what we have for you," Carol says.

"What is it?" asks Jay.

"Bagels from South Florida. Every kind you can think of, onion, poppy seed..." She goes on. "I'll bring them up in awhile. We need to unload right now. See you later."

Once inside I separate bagels into bags of five for neighbors. Then Carol makes her deliveries, while I fix a light meal. I think of the day while heating food, and hope these new pills will cure her. When she's back, we sit for dinner, saying grace first. Carol takes two little white pills. My silent prayer, *"Please cure her."*

5

In the weeks ahead, we walk the beach, play golf, walk the heart trail—two and a half miles worth, ride bikes in the neighborhood after dinner and swim in the pool in the mornings as usual. My thought now is: we exercised all the time to keep the body in good physical shape, so it wouldn't break down. *Why then has this happened? Why is the disease here?*

For my birthday, Carol takes me to the golf club she belongs. The exclusive one she came to for six months while living up north, years before I knew her. She's made the decision now to drop the membership.

St. Patty's Day comes, and we join neighbors at the condo club house. We dress in green and white, enjoying a dinner of corned beef and cabbage and green Jell-O for dessert. Things are good.

Days later, a friend of Carol's dies, and she asks if I'll take her to the memorial service. I watch as she talks to her friends, telling them she has Alzheimer's. Again, I'm amazed at how open she is about her illness. I'm not, and feel there is a stain placed upon her.

Joeie, my neighbor from St. James, and Carla, Carol's golf friend come to join us for golf and lunch. My friend Joeie, and her husband, have bought a condo just north of us. In golf carts we ride; Joeie with me, and Carla with Carol. At the end of our match, Carol adds up scores, saying she has trouble seeing, but I know she's having trouble adding.

When done we go home for lunch instead of eating out. I had prepared a meal the day before and there is little left to do. Joeie and I toss a salad in the kitchen, while Carla and Carol sit on the porch.

"She's different, Rose," Joeie says.

"What do you mean?"

"She's changed since I last saw her. Her look is different. She doesn't have that soft smile anymore. She looks worried, and thinner."

I wonder what Carla's thinking, since she's known her for many years, on the Island and in Florida.

"I guess I don't see it, because I'm around her every day. I don't know what I'm going to do without her, Joeie."

She puts her arm around me saying, "She still plays a great golf game, but she's not the old Carol I remember."

"I guess we better call them in, before the carrot soup simmers down to nothing. Thanks for coming Joeie, it's great to see you again."

"It's good to see you too, my friend."

I still remember that first day I saw Carol coming up the eighteenth fairway, with those long legs. I'd asked Joeie who she was, and she'd told me she was the best golfer on the Island.

***

Carol's doing taxes and wants me to learn. "It's Greek," I tell her. "I've never done anything like this." Carol, like Ed, had handled all household finances. When she had made me power of attorney and health care advocate in '86, I wanted no part of it. Nothing was going to happen to her, if anything, I'd drop dead before her. She had been a Girl Scout, taught to plan for everything. *Me?* I hoped for the best and never planned for anything. I figured God would get me through whatever it was. Blind faith, you might say. She wanted to put the condo in both our names, but my divorce attorney said, 'no, it would be personal property and Ed would be entitled to half.' So Carol put the condo in her name, willing it to me upon her death, like the pussy willows she had promised Hope, except this was real. Ed had life insurance policies and mutual funds but handled all of it at work. We were husband and wife. If anyone died the other would inherit, simple. My divorce is moving slow because he's still dragging his feet and not cooperating. I tell my attorney, "Do whatever is necessary, I want it over with." My attorney assures me, the settlement will take care of me for life, and not to worry about money. I don't. I worry about Carol.

She teaches me financial statements; how entries are made on paper, monies accumulated and what goes out to pay bills. She teaches me dividends, monthly, quarterly, yearly, where to pencil them in on the sheet she'd made. Out of this, comes the yearly income, which needs to be sent to the accountant for taxes. It's hard. But she sits week after week teaching me at the dining room table. She's preparing me, but I don't want to learn this part of our relationship. I want to enjoy life, with her.

Our next research visit I tell Dr. Mike I'm learning household finances, and don't get it. "Get a computer and a program called 'financial builder'," he says, "You'll be able to track investments and bills."

So, a computer is delivered, which neither of us know anything about. I read step by step instructions and start recording investments and bills. It's easier punching keys than writing it down. Carol continues her way and we compare at the end of the month. I watch the stock market on television, learning how the economy works. I hated money and what it did to people, especially my father. He'd been cheap, while his wife worked her heart out. The arguments they had were always over money. Then there was Ed, and his money. Money left a sour taste in my mouth. Now, I have no choice, I have to learn how it affects one's life.

While on the drug, Carol has stomach discomfort, trying different soothers for indigestion.

We travel to Tamarac once a month for cognitive testing. Dr. Mike asks me how she's doing at home. "I don't see any difference, except for her dizziness in the morning before eating, and she still leaves things out of place around the house. Other than that, we're playing golf and she's doing her chores, just a little slower."

I receive a call from Mom saying she needs surgery to remove part of her colon. She has cancer. I speak with her doctor and my brothers afterward, finding the operation went well and they'll reattach her colon in six months.

I feel bad not being there with her, but know Paul and Marc are close by, and John is there for her. We'll get back to our daily phone calls when she's better.

In May, Carol's given a new drug because of her stomach reaction to Nimo.

Am I losing hope? Is Carol losing hope?

We don't talk of it and keep an 'up' feeling between us. My feelings are if we don't talk about it, it won't be there.

I make reservations at the Dora Golf Resort for two days, as it's not far from the research center. I remember being there with Ed, years ago. I wasn't into golf back then, but this will be a nice surprise for Carol, she's never been there. Plus we will have something to look forward to after our clinic visit.

When we arrive, I remember the brass railings leading up the brick steps. A valet parks the car, and we go inside. I give the woman behind the desk our names, and she sends for a bellhop to take us to our room. I look at Carol a few times and see happiness.

"The room is beautiful. I love the colors," she says. It's large with cheerful colors of light blue and yellow, her favorite.

"C'mon, Ca, let's change, and play nine holes." There's no discussion. She's ready when I come out of the bathroom.

"Boy that was fast. How'd you get dressed so fast?"

"You said the word *golf*. I love to play this time of the day, shadows on the greens."

Late afternoon *was* the best time to play, empty course and a cool breeze. We kid with our usual match of one up or one down or tied. This time we are not playing for who is going to cook dinner, which was always a laugh, because she didn't cook anyway. We're just happy.

After taking showers, we sit near open French doors eating dinner. A kitten appears and Carol speaks to it and like all animals, it comes to her. She tells the waiter the kitty is hungry. While having dessert, the kitten gets her milk.

I look across the table, see the softness back on her face, and ask her, "You having fun, Ca?"

"Oh yes! It's a lovely place, and the golf course is great. Are *you* having fun?"

"I sure am. Wait till you see the championship course tomorrow—you're gonna love it. Ed and I were here in the 60s. Just watching you makes *my* fun."

After a day of play the next day, we sit on the open patio overlooking the course, sipping lemonade, going over scorecards.

"Well, it's not too bad," I say. "We both shot in the eighties, but I beat you by four shots." These days were rare in our past games. I never beat the best golfer of Long Island, there or anywhere else. Seeing something beautiful, I say, "Look behind you, Ca. See the impatiens hanging on the trees. Isn't that a brilliant idea? Maybe we could do that in our courtyard?"

"It *is* pretty."

We sit outside until the sun starts its decline, enjoying the greenery and watching birds search for their dinner in ponds. Afterward, seated in the same dining room, at the same table as the night before, with the same kitten, we see she has her milk. Later, we walk the complex looking in shops, enjoying each other's company. It's been a glorious day. Carol's made me feel connected.

A month later, we are back at the research center, same testing with the same people. Carol takes off to one office, I to another, and we meet later. While waiting for her, I see a man who's been here before. He comes with his wife and tells me she was a songwriter years ago and can't remember anything now. He mentions songs she's published, but I'm not familiar with them. He's eighty. I'm at the end of my forties. I see in his eyes what I'm sure he sees in mine—fear of losing a loved one.

Dr. Mike calls me in while Carol's in another room. "Carol didn't do well on the tests," he says. "She dropped a few points."

"Oh?" I hear, but don't want to.

Carol comes in, all smiles, "C'mon, let's get something to eat, I'm starving." She has that bouncy look about her, full of energy.

I look at Dr. Mike, and he gives the okay. "See you next month," he says.

Together, we say, "Goodbye."

We stop to eat, then bagels for neighbors, as usual. The drive is longer than usual and Carol falls asleep. I have my own thoughts to go over on this drive. I'm not joyous. I just don't know what to think anymore. But I do know what I heard at the center. 'Carol didn't do well on the tests.'

6

Hey, girls, let me treat you to dinner."

October 16, 1991, my brother Marc is here. Seeing his face is great, but having another in the household is even nicer. We've been talking for hours in the living room and Carol has excused herself to use the bathroom.

"We'll see," I say. "How are the kids?" I ask. Marc has five children, all adults now.

"Good, everyone's fine. They're all doing their own thing. Between school and work, I never know what they're up to. Thank God they don't give me any trouble. So, where do you want to eat tonight?"

"There's a place around the corner that has great seafood. I think you'll like it. If we leave soon, we can catch the 'early bird' special. Let's see what Carol thinks."

"Sounds great. I eat fish all the time since my cholesterol's high. I gotta watch my waistline, you know," he smiles. He had a heart attack in his early fifties, but you'd never know it to look at him. He's slender, keeps himself fit playing golf and tennis, and still works as a pharmacist.

"You look great—too bad I don't take after you." I had a potbelly, I wasn't proud of. Keeping Carol and myself happy in ice cream, had become a steady diet.

"So where are we going for dinner?" Carol asks, returning.

"I thought we'd take Marc to Harpon Harry's. What do you think?"

"Good idea. Food's good, and he should like the scenery."

Harpon Harry's was the first restaurant she'd taken me to in 1985, when we dressed in blue blazers. Seeing our reflections in an elevator mirror, I had said she was the taller one, and she said, 'no, you're the shorter one.' Now, *Marc* is fascinated by the red light house, across the waterway, taking pictures. He's tried his hand at photography and explains, after a few martinis, what his camera can do. I think, *it probably can walk and take it's own pictures after his long explanation.*

The next day we show Marc around town ride up Jupiter Island, where the elite live. In the backseat, he says, "Everyone's looking at me."

"What are you talking about? Who's looking at you?" I ask.

"Don't you see the car next to us? They're looking at me." Carol and I check the car next to us.

"No one's looking at you, Marc."

"Sure they are. They're wondering who I am, being chauffeured by two gorgeous women."

I laugh. Carol stifles hers. "He's a great guy, this brother of mine—always full of compliments."

During his visit, we play golf, and Carol teaches him the finer points of the game.

"Hold the club like a baby bird," she says, "and swing like a rag doll."

The same tips I heard long ago. Marc knows they're coming from the best. His company makes us forget our troubles.

Carol walks to the lobby to get the mail and Marc asks me, "What are you going to do with her?"

"What do you mean, what am I going to do with her? I'm going to take care of her like I promised."

"Are you crazy? Do you know what you're in for? She's changed a lot, Rose."

"I know she's changed. Let's not go into it. I've made up my mind to care for her, and that's what I'll do. You forget how much she did for me."

Carol had taken me in after I'd left Ed and the kids on Long Island. She'd treated me like family, helped me believe in myself, helped me learn to live without fear and depression. I owed her more than my life.

Four days later Marc drives south to Ft. Lauderdale and Miami. I hate saying goodbye and have no idea when I'll see him or any of my family again. I miss them.

It's been a year since the diagnosis, and I notice Carol's writing less in her little black daily entry books. She no longer tapes words to my mirror for me to learn and improve my vocabulary, but I do read the writing she taped inside my cabinet years ago. *Don't look forward to what might happen tomorrow. The same everlasting Father who cares for you today will care for you tomorrow and everyday. Either He will shield you from suffering, or He will give you unfailing strength to bear it. Be at peace and put away all anxious thoughts.* I try hard not to look forward.

Thanksgiving, we invite neighbors. Christmas is different; we go to a Methodist church at eight o'clock, instead of our traditional Catholic midnight-mass. It's easier, she doesn't have to remember, sit, stand, kneel. We decorate a tree, exchange one present before bedtime.

A new year begins playing nine holes instead of eighteen. Days are filled with doctors and research. I search the Internet for answers, but little is written on Alzheimer's. We swim, and walk the heart path when we're not at medical offices. Our lives of yesterday have come to a halt. Each morning is illness. She's getting worse by the minute.

I buy a Tai Chi video for exercise; she stands behind me, following my moves. Everyday I say, "Now your arms, Ca. Up, down, to the side. Now, let's work on the legs. Lift them high Ca, like walking up stairs." She tries, but it's hard for her. I can't let her stop everything. We attend the Alzheimer's support group every week coming home more depressed, hearing stories, how the disease robs the brain. I make milkshakes with ice cream and bananas, so she won't lose more weight. The doctor says her brain is shutting down. I don't believe him.

I can't let *it* get her.

7

Summer 1992, just shy of two years after diagnosis, Dr. Mike switches Carol to the Italian study. She's having heart palpitations every morning. We don't need to make the trip south every month. Now, it's every third month. She likes the idea, she's won't get stuck with needles as often. *A good thing.*

I take it on myself to rent a house on Long Island for three months, one block from where Carol lived with her parents. At first I think I'll surprise her, then think it might not be a good idea and decide to tell her. Her words have decreased and I think seeing old friends and places might help. She likes the idea.

"Sounds good," she says.

Hope is having her first child and wants me there for the birth. When she married last year, I couldn't be there, so now I'll spend time with her firstborn. Matthew is married with two children, and I can't wait to see them. The children and life, have gotten away from me. Renting a house, they'll be able to visit, maybe stay over.

Getting out the door is harried, but soon we are on our way for the two and a half hour drive to the auto train.

Carol looks out the window, making comments of fast traffic and trees. I've brought 'books on tape' along to occupy our minds. In Winter Park, we grab a snack before boarding the four-thirty train. It's shorter by nine hundred miles, and fun meeting other travelers.

The next morning at eight-thirty, we're in Virginia. I've decided to drive to Connecticut to see Helen and David, friends of Carol's mother. They've known her since she was a baby and I see how much they love her. While David cooks, Helen sets the table. "Let us help," I say. Helen says, 'no, tell us of Florida.'

Carol has kept up with them, calling on holidays, writing birthday and anniversary cards. She had written them of her Alzheimer's when she wrote others after she'd been diagnosed. She amazed me then when she did it. But then, she's always amazed me.

Carol gets up to go to the bathroom and can't find it, so I help her look. I think to myself, this is a house she'd been many times before and now she can't find the bathroom? Helen calls me aside when I go back to the kitchen.

"She's really gone, isn't she?"

"No—she's changed, but she's still the same old Carol. She just has trouble getting her words together," I say, hurting for my friend.

My thought? They hate seeing her decline, like me.

We sleep in the guest bedroom, with a joining bathroom that night. A room with two four-poster beds, high off the floor. Carol's tall, and has no problem getting in bed. I need a stool—two steps up, and I sink deep into feathers.

"Hey, Ca, can you see me?" I ask, sucked up by the mattress. "I feel like I'm in a hole." And we laugh.

53

In the middle of the night, I get up to use the bathroom, and fall on my knees, forgetting to use the stool.

"Are you hurt?"

"No, I'm fine, but remind me never to buy a bed of feathers."

The next day, saying goodbye, Helen takes Carol by the hand and leads her to the curio cabinet filled with cut and colored glass.

"Pick anything you want," Helen says.

Carol reaches for the glass bluebird.

"The bluebird of happiness, it's yours."

Pulling away from the tucked in the woods, Connecticut home, we wave, me knowing it's Carol's last visit. I ache for her and them. *Maybe blue bird will help her.*

The trip to St. James isn't bad, only three hours. We stop first at Mom's apartment. I had told her we were coming, but not the exact time. I knock. John opens the door.

"Oh, look who's here! Maria—Maria, come quickly."

I hear Mom in the kitchen, "Who's here, Santa Claus?"

Creeping up behind her, cooking, "Hi, Mom." and surprise her. At a loss for words, she wraps her arms around me. I hold her. Then she sees Carol, and hugs her. An image of Mutt and Jeff, from old newspaper funnies, crosses my mind.

"Stay for dinner."

"No, Mom. It's been a long trip, and I want to see the house before it gets dark."

"I'm glad you're here. It'll be good for you to rest."

"The house is ten minutes away, so we can visit anytime. I'll call you tomorrow."

Stony Brook is a small town on the north shore and I'd taken Matthew and Hope fishing with Mom on summer days, or just Mom and I would have lunch in the small café. Approaching now, I'm happy with memories here, and see Carol's face beaming and hear it in her voice. She knows.

"The country store," she says.

"Yeah, and the ice cream parlor, right next door. Yippee. How about we get chicken salad for dinner, and ice cream?"

"Okay."

She recognizes it. I know she does. *New hope.* Maybe this *is* what she needs, her hometown again.

We pull up to the ranch house, *pretty.* Decorated similar to Carol's parents' home; pictures she'd showed me. The Williamsburg look, mahogany furniture, printed fabrics on chairs, and window treatments. *She should feel right at home.* One room has twin beds. We'll make it our room.

She doesn't say much going from room to room, just smiles a lot. I'm happy.

While having dinner, I ask, "It's a nice house, isn't it, Ca?"

"Yes, I like it."

"You know, it's around the corner from your old house."

"I know the people across the street."

"Really? Maybe we can visit them. What's their name?"

She thinks hard, and then says, "I can't remember."

"I wonder if they still live there?"

55

She says nothing.

When finished, we throw the garbage outside. It's warm out, and a fragrance in the air as we walk up the street. I miss the Island's flowers, rhododendrons, azaleas, tulips, dogwood and cherry tree blossoms. *Maybe she does, too.* The houses are mostly colonials, with manicured lawns. They have pebble driveways. *I miss this look.*

Later, we change into nightwear. "I'll sleep near the door," I tell her. She gets into the other bed. I open a book, read a page then hear her snoring, and turn off the light. It's been a long day.

I wake in the middle of the night hearing sounds. Her bed's empty. "Ca. Where are you?" I call, and check the bathroom in the hall. Not there, and call again.

I find her in the kitchen turning the water faucet on and off, mumbling. Fear is on her face for the fist time, similar to my own terror that I remember. I put my arm around her and ask, "Do you want a drink?"

She nods. I fill a glass halfway with water.

"It's all right, Ca. In a few days, you'll be right at home. You wait and see. Do you need to use the bathroom?"

She nods faster. I realize then, she *was* looking for the bathroom. Compassion fills me.

When finished, I lead her back to bed. The next night is the same, and the night after that, and the night after that. I decide the den will be our home base, since it has an adjoining bathroom and sofa bed.

We visit her old house and meet the owners. Before leaving Florida she had packed old pictures of the house and vacant land it was built on. She thought the owners might like to have them. I thought it was a good idea. Now, they look at photos, happy she's brought them. They're interested in the house, how it came to be, and ask questions. They serve tea, and I watch her go into great detail of home fires her father built, and when the swan smacked her mother with its wings, when she had gone down to the pond one day. She speaks of her parents mostly, even her grandmother, Chris, who lived with them after her stroke. She tells of the portrait that hung over the fireplace that now hangs in our home.

I listen, feeling this is the old Carol, deciding it *was* a good idea to bring her back.

But how is it she remembers this and doesn't remember where the bathroom is?

In September we watch The Ladies Club Championship, and remember our last match in '85. We invite friends and family for dinners and watch birds at the feeder every morning, assigning them names. It's like old times, but Hope is the only one who declines our invites. We go to brother Marc's home where Mom makes dinner while Marc teases her of too much salt in the tomato sauce. Carol, Marc's children and I sit laughing at the bantering between mother and son. "Marc, listen to your mother," I say.

The vacation is good, but late afternoons and nights are chaotic. She's up, out of bed heading for the bathroom all hours of the night and having trouble finding the right words to say to me or anyone else. I see her embarrassment when she stops mid sentence in conversation, not able to find the right word. We go to dinner with family, she gets upset, excusing herself from the table. I find her in the bathroom wringing her hands, knowing she is *not* all right. She can't tell me what's wrong.

Something else is wrong. This isn't her. Can it be the Italian study medication? I call Dr. Mike. He says it could be but not likely. Maybe we should see a doctor. We visit her former Long Island doctor. He finds a urinary tract infection, says this could account for her confusion, constant trips to the bathroom, and not being herself. Thank God—an answer.

A month and a half into the trip, she's no better on antibiotics, and her confusion is worse. I've called Hope everyday wanting to see her, have a cup of coffee, talk of old times, just see her face. But everyday I hear the same, 'not today'. She hasn't had the baby yet, and I worry about her. She doesn't sound like the Hope I once knew. She doesn't ask of Carol, or how she's doing and doesn't seem to care. This is the child who loved Carol, more than her own mother, sometimes I thought. Discouraged and hurt, I want to go home.

8

Back home is harder. Carol is depressed, something new.

"I can't *do* anything!" she cries.

"Yes, you can," feeling the pain with her.

"No, I can't—I hate this! I can't do paperwork— I'm useless!"

I take her hand, "No—no, you're not. I don't want to hear that. You write birthday and anniversary cards. I don't—*you* do." I'd made it easier for her by typing names and dates on the computer then printing them for her. "We do the bills and investments together. I wouldn't know how to do it if it weren't for you. Please don't be upset."

I try convincing her she's not useless by drying dishes, sweeping the patio, and other jobs around the house that she *can* do. I want her to keep busy.

My hands are tied, I know. I can only help a little. It's the medical profession that can really help. She sits at her desk with papers, me thinking she's working on something, then find her crying.

"I'm losing my mind. I can't think anymore," she tells me.

"You're not losing your mind. The medicine is going to help. You wait and see—it will."

Am I fooling myself and her? But I need something to go on. *We* need something to believe in.

She calms down, and I end up in my bathroom crying, because it hurts so. She was never depressed. She was always up on life. She found the good in everything, even if it was negative to someone else.

The support group says, 'It's just a stage and will leave soon.' My question, "what are we going to find in the next stage?"

How can she be so near in body, yet so far in mind?

Moments of happiness come when I hear chirping, "Ca, Geech is here get the seeds." And she runs for the sunflower seeds. She puts them on the table in front of the kitchen window where we watch. I never thought this little red bird would be such a gift. I think it only yesterday when she named the cardinal after her uncle, but it isn't. It's been years.

At the end of 1992, we're living each day as it comes not looking to the future. It seems all dark ahead of us.

Something new has started.

"What time is it?" she asks.

"It's 3 o'clock," I answer.

A few seconds later, "What time is it?"

"It's 3 o'clock."

"What time is it?"

"Ca—it's 3 o'clock, I just told you a minute ago."

Forgetting, she asks over and over, driving *me* crazy. The support group lets me know, we are not the only ones going through this terrible time. So, I learn to let it go in

60

one ear and out the other, but wonder, *Why is it she remembers the question and doesn't remember the answer?*

I lie to her so she won't become agitated and I can keep my sanity. Making a simple mistake, like telling her we're going to the research center tomorrow, will keep us up all night. "When are we going? When are we going?" she asks, and looks in her black book or a note she's scribbled on a piece of paper on her desk. She's forgotten all concept of time. I learn not to tell her until it's time to do anything we have to do.

Today is the first day I've had the desire to write. I've thought about it for months, even years, but this is the first I feel the need. I want to write of the struggle she's going through with this horrific disease; the everyday living. I want to write how the caregiver loses herself along with the victim. *Victim*—first time I've ever used that word. But there's no other word that best describes it. After all she is a victim of time.

I've lost any thought that she'll get better. I've come to the conclusion I'm living alone, even though she's with me in body. She doesn't talk to me in an understandable conversation. We play charades to discover what she wants.

I've stopped all walks and exercise. My agoraphobia is back or has it just been hiding? I don't want to go to the store because I'm alone, even though she's at my side. I hate life, eating fatty foods, hoping to bring on a heart attack and die. Then I won't have to face her dying in front of me, inch by inch.

I thought she understood what she read, until one night I asked her to tell me the newspaper article she was reading. "Oh, you know, you know," she said, flailing her arms about. I realized then she *didn't* understand what she read and gave up on any miracle.

The same night I asked, "Ca, are you happy?"

She shrugged, motioning toward heaven, as if to say, 'Yes, what else can I be? I can't do anything about it.'

Those pretty much were her words, as I perceived, and I thought, *she's still happy, leaving it all up to God's plan.* She takes whatever life offers her. She's a greater person than I could ever hope to be. I wish though, I didn't remember what she was like before. I saw her talk to the butterflies and lizards outside our condo. She whispered to flowers so they would grow healthy and feel loved. Some people thought she was nuts back then. Not me. I knew she was a part of nature, God's creation. A pure child of God.

I'm up against a brick wall and can't do a thing except make sure she's clean and fed.

Thanksgiving and Christmas came and left, we didn't even know.

She walks constantly for no reason and her weight's gone from 175 to 130, almost over night. She looks ill. Her rib cage shows, I see her spine and can count each vertebra. Dr. Mike and Dr. Ban ask me if she's eating.

"Yes, she's eating everything in sight," I say.

Again Dr. Ban says the brain is shutting down. I make shakes and order choline from the drugstore. I've read it's good for the brain. I can't believe the doctor. *I can make her better.*

She gains weight, and I feel better. The urinary problem improves. I remind her to use the bathroom every two hours and drink cranberry juice*, there's hope.*

It's March 21, 1993. I don't want to write today. I'm mad, and lonely. I miss my friend. Carol isn't really here anymore.

"Where is Rose?" I ask her.

"She's here," she utters words (not those) and motions with her hands and arms. I decipher she means, "Rose is around here somewhere."

But, how can that be when I'm standing right in front of her? Why doesn't she say, 'SHE'S RIGHT HERE.' Maybe she doesn't remember me.

I bring her down on the research pills, there's a new pill coming out that shows promise. I'm playing with a life—to give a pill? or not to give a pill? The new drug has helped people mentally and physically in research.

I read in the newspaper a man shoots his wife who had Alzheimer's. *Could I do this?*

Why doesn't the government help? Drugs must be passed sooner for a cure. Money goes for beautiful offices and trips made by CEOs. I've never felt this way about my country, but watching her decline, and knowing I won't have health insurance after my divorce, has changed my thoughts.

I see terror on her face and it reminds me of my panic attacks. I stay close to her, letting her know she's not alone. I'll always be there for her. I'm no doctor, but I know what she feels, I'm living with her 24/7. She's never out of sight.

Lately she doesn't want to come to the table to eat. So I bribe her, saying, "No chocolate pudding or chocalotta ice cream if you don't finish your dinner." Like raising my children. She likes sweets all the time; yet when she was well, she rarely ate them, except ice cream. *The brain has to be craving sugar for a reason.* I buy a juicer, make fresh vegetable and fruit juices, because a man on TV says it will make the body strong and healthy.

So many chores to do: clean the house, paper work, trying to keep her clean. She changes clothes in the middle of the night, putting clothes on top of clothes. I sleep with her, rubbing her arm, to calm her. Around two in the morning, she stirs, fiddling with her clothes. I leave, and go to my room for rest. The burglar alarm is set. She can't go out without me hearing. I need sleep if I'm going to care for her. Her hair is falling out for no obvious reason, black circles are under her eyes. She doesn't yawn anymore when she's tired. Strange, and I think and wonder if other victims do this? The doctors have no answers. I wish something else would show in tests. I wish she had cancer instead of this disease of losing her mind. She's sliding fast, like a runaway train. There's no stopping it. I hate this disease. All I want to do is comfort her.

9

By July '93, we're shopping at the dinner hour when the store is empty. Carol pushes the cart. I pull.

"We need cereal, Ca. Get shredded wheat. I'll get oatmeal." She reaches for the yellow box, puts it in the basket. I grab oatmeal.

This is our exercise, walking from aisle to aisle. We're out—somewhere different from the walls we've come to know so well.

Home from the store I see a stain on the dining room ceiling. She's gone to her bedroom to pace, her new habit now. The support group calls it *sundowners*. I find the room behind the dining room also has a stain. I call Jay upstairs, ask him to check his floor for wetness. He tells me to hang on, then comes back saying, "No, nothing here. Maybe it's the seal under your toilet. We've replaced a number of them the past few years. I'll come down and check."

I thank him and hang up. Carol has come into the dining room when Jay arrives.

"Oh, that's a pretty big stain," he says and goes to check the bathroom seal. It's okay. He puts his ear to the dining room wall. "Uh oh…sounds like you have a leak. Come, listen."

I put my ear to the wall and hear dripping inside. "Oh God Jay, like we really need this, now?"

As the night goes on, I learn Jay's rug is wet under the organ and other neighbors above us have wet rugs. I call the plumber. Everyone coming in and out of the condo, Carol retreats to her bedroom to pace and talk to herself. Everyone looks to me for an answer.

"She'll be all right. She's just upset seeing so many people." I go for the chocolate chip cookies, give them to her and she smiles that beautiful smile.

The plumber tells us to shut off our main water valves and he'll be back in the morning to check the roof. When I say goodnight to all, the stains are larger, now in three rooms.

I wake in the middle of the night to the sound of water rushing down from the ceiling into the bathtub. Checking the dining room, living room and guest bedroom, I walk through a carpet swamp.

By daylight, the plumber and neighbors have gathered on the roof. I call the insurance company.

The plumber says a drainpipe was closed by mistake, when the new roof was put on three years ago.

The condo insurance will cover it, and our private insurance will cover the inside. Thank God.

I make phone calls while Carol paces through the 'swamp', agitated. Our insurance company gives me the name of a contractor who says, we'll never get rid of the damage. "You're gonna need new rugs and walls," he says. Insurance agrees to pay ninety percent of remodeling fees.

Workers come and Carol's impossible to handle. Having too many people in the house at one time, she runs outside every chance she gets. A door opens for a worker, she runs out before it's closed. I run after her. I call the nearest motel for a room that we can call home for awhile. I dress her every morning, to meet the workers at the condo letting them in, then go back to the motel. At four-thirty it's back to the condo locking up when workers leave.

Carpet is ripped up, walls broken through. Workers lift a credenza, and the bottom falls off. A heavy piece, we never moved—rotted wood. *How long has it been like this?* The molding behind the piece has doubled in size. When the workers break through the wall, I see colored mold—black, red, and white dots. The water has been there for years a worker says. Under Carol's file cabinet, carpet is soaked, covered with black mold—another piece we never touched since moving in.

Her confusion is worse, and mine isn't far behind. At the grocery store buying items to bring back to the motel, we wait at the deli counter for turkey sandwiches. I hear, "Hello, you two." Bob, our old neighbor from the ocean condo.

"Hi, long time, no see."

Carol smiles.

"What are you up to? I haven't seen you in so long, I thought you left town."

"We live at Garden Parks. Carol bought a place in '86. How's your diabetes? Is it still acting up, or are you eating all the right foods now?" I ask, grinning, because Bob never ate the right foods. Living next to Carol years ago when she was down on vacation for six months, Bob threw great parties. When Hope and her friends came for a visit, he took them fishing. He was a good neighbor and friend we'd lost contact with. Carol liked Bob back then, now she can't say anything to him.

I whisper to him while she's looking at something on the shelf, "She has Alzheimer's."

"Oh no...I thought something was wrong when she didn't say hello."

An idea comes to me, "Bob, is there anything for rent in your building?"

"My neighbor won't be down this year. Her husband died on February fourteenth."

Funny, Carol's birthday.

I excuse myself and run after Carol who's headed for the outside door. The one split second I turned to talk, she's gone. Now I take her hand and lead her back to Bob.

"Do me a favor Bob, see if your neighbor will rent the place to us. You know we're good tenants and won't destroy it. We had a flood and are staying at the motel across the bridge." I write the motel number on the back of a piece of paper, and hand it to him.

"You take care now. I'll call you tonight. Bye, Carol," he says, and in my amazement, she waves.

The lady behind the counter hands me sandwiches and we go to our favorite place, the inlet, to watch the boats and eat lunch.

Bob calls at eight-thirty saying to meet him at the condo in the morning.

After a motel buffet breakfast, we go to Sea Trail. Bob buzzes us in the front door. We take the elevator to the third floor. I hold under her arm in case she gets confused and wants to run. I have no idea how she'll act, being inside the same building she used to winter in, years ago.

Walking the catwalk to #305, she holds me back. "It's okay. C'mon, Ca. Everything's all right."

I see Bob standing at the door, watching us.

Inside it's dark, hurricane shutters closed across the balcony, stopping outside light from entering.

"Bob, will you please open the shutters?"

He rolls them back and the ocean comes into full view. "Ohoooo…," Carol says, and her long strides pull me with her.

I hold back tears, knowing my friend has come alive, as she leads me to the balcony. *She's happy.*

"Well Bob, I guess we'll take it. I think Carol just made the decision."

We lean over the balcony watching the ocean and people below swimming in the pool. I talk with Bob and watch my friend. It's *all* so beautiful.

"Bob, when do you think we can move in? It's awful living at the motel."

"I'll talk to the president of the board. There shouldn't be a problem since she's lived here before."

"Thank you, Robert. You're a God send."

When it's time to leave I take her hand, but she doesn't budge. "We're coming back, Ca—I promise," and finally she lets me lead her.

Later that day, after getting some things from home, I sit on the balcony overlooking the blue-green water while my friend lays on the lounge gazing at the ocean. *She's content.* It's going to cost a lot, but her lawyer said, 'Do anything that makes her happy.' And from the smile on her face, I'd say she's happy.

I give the key to our home to the contractor, so I won't have to let him in every morning. The work is going well, but will take months before the place is livable. No matter now, we have another home for a year.

I hang her portrait over the couch. It belongs here. She enjoys lying outside on the balcony, instead of pacing. We eat breakfast, lunch, and dinner outside as we did years ago when I came from the unhappiness up north. We swim in the pool, walk the beach and our skin goes from a sickly white to beautiful bronze. She looks *almost* healthy.

10

This morning is a morning only God could have made. The air is warm, and a breeze kisses your cheeks, feeling like velvet. We are going for an ocean swim, for the first time. Carol's in first, the better swimmer, and swims out. I stay in the shallow water. I watch the stroke I've seen for years, elbows point out, head in the water then out for breath, she glides as a fish. But, she's out too far. I can't save her if anything happens. Fear comes, and I yell, "Ca, come back! You're out too far!" She doesn't hear. Cupping my hands to my mouth, I yell louder, "Ca, come back here. GET BACK HERE RIGHT NOW!"

She turns, smiles and waves, as if to say, 'I'm all right, it's fun.'

Should I tell the lifeguard? Then see she's turned swimming towards me. Just like watching my children when they were young. Now *she's* my child. The thought bothers me.

Close now, she splashes me. "Cut it out. Don't you dare go out that far again. You stay with me. I can't swim in water over my head, you know that." She nods, as if she does know.

Later, we walk the wooden path through the dunes, as years before, except this time, I have hold of her hand, leading her to the tar station.

"Sit down, Ca. I need to clean your feet." A bench had been put there to sit, in order to remove tar from ones feet. Ocean barges have a habit of spilling small amounts of oil that wash up on shore and mix with sand.

I reach for the mineral spirits and cloth to clean her feet. Bending down, out of the corner of my eye I see a woman standing. "We're going to be a while, so if you want to use the hose, go ahead," I say.

"No, that's okay. I'm in no hurry. I'll wait."

I reach my hand out, "Hi, I'm Rose. This is Carol. We're in 305."

"Hi, I'm Debbi. I'm on the 10th floor. Nice to meet you."

I rub Carol's feet free of tar. "We moved in a week ago. It's amazing how much tar you pick up out there. Carol used to live here in winter months."

I'm sure Debbi's wondering why Carol isn't joining in the conversation. I see Carol reading our faces. If she sees doubt, she'll react with fear and run. I don't want that.

"Ready to go?" I say, reaching for Carol's hand. "Goodbye, Debbi. It was nice to meet you."

"Bye. Good to have you back, Carol."

She smiles at Debbi. She does know what people say to her.

In the days and weeks ahead, I find Debbi is a psychotherapist and tell her of Carol's illness. I explain our living conditions and she offers her help. Giving me books on encouragement and faith, she tells me if I need to talk, she'll help in any way she can. I can't thank her enough, because Carol and I have become loners, except for Bob who stops in once in a while to say hello. I've found, because of the illness, people talk around it or make believe it doesn't exist. Friends have told me they will call but never do. We've been abandoned.

Carol is happy living at the ocean, so am I. We enjoy the shorebirds, and the smell of clean, fresh, salt air. She's been on a new drug for a couple of months, one passed by the FDA for Alzheimer's. At first, she took ten milligrams, and has slowly worked up to forty, four times a day. There's a difference, I can see it. She's more alert, and washes herself. She's reading again but can't speak in sentences. I don't understand why, but she's better.

11

Mom has had a heart attack and is being transferred to a New York City hospital, where she will have bypass surgery. For years I have spoken with her every Sunday but now I call her several times a day to talk. I know we won't talk again until after the operation and she's recuperating. "Mom, I love you," I say. "You know I'm not there in body, but I'm with you in spirit." I want to be with her, but can't, I have Carol.

"Yes, I know. I love you, too. You take good care of yourself," she says. "It's an adventure if I make it, and an adventure if I don't."

After other words of comfort, I tell her I'll talk with her in a few days, when she's able, holding back my own tears.

Two days later Paul calls telling me Mom has passed of a massive stroke. The conversation with him is short, and in tears I make my way to the balcony. Carol stops pacing and follows me. Her hands hold my face. She's sad, her eyes have tears also, and I feel the words '*I'm sorry*,' not spoken, but I know I hear them.

"It's okay, Ca. Mom's with God now," and she keeps me company on the balcony for a while until her agitation calls her to pace once again.

Carol's improvement doesn't last. I prayed it would and that she'd even get better, or even cured, but that didn't happen. Christmas is very different this year. I place a two-foot fake tree, already decorated, on a table, and cook a simple meal. It's memorable, but for other reasons. We attend Christmas Day mass, and she can't sit through the service, so we leave. I hate the thought of losing her. Every morning, I wake not believing what's happened—she has a disease that rids her of her dignity and being. It's getting harder and harder.

12

In the corner of the dining room, stands a large plant, mostly green leaves with little white flowers. I notice the flowers are getting less and less. Sitting on the couch, I watch her pace from room to room. She stops at the plant, and picks a flower.

I tell her, "please, don't pick the flowers. It's not our plant." She looks at me, then the flower, mimics me and then throws the flower behind the plant. I get up and find twenty others in the same corner. *What goes through her mind when she does this? Does she think they're real?*

I haven't written in my so called diary for quite a while. *I'm* getting bouts of confusion. Maybe I'm getting Alzheimer's? Doctor says, 'no, it's only depression.'

It's almost ten years, and still I have no divorce. Ed fights me on everything. He doesn't want to share any of *his* assets. My attorney says his lawyer doesn't return any calls, and I need to be in New York to fight the case. *Great, something more to think about.*

Six months gone so fast, and I don't know where the days go. This day Carol's on the balcony and waves for me to come. She can't say the words, *'Come here'* but moves her hands beckoning me, speaking in another language, I've come to understand some.

"Rah, Rah, Rah," she says softly.

I join her.

"What, Ca? What is it?"

"Rah, Rah, Rah," she says, pointing.

Leaning over the balcony, I see nothing and then in the trellis directly below, I see a nest holding a pair of doves.

"Oh, look at that. I see it, Ca."

"Rah, Rah."

"Yes, I see them."

She's excited. I'm excited, my friend has spotted nature, again.

We go to the balcony everyday watching the progress of two workers. Soon eggs are in the nest. I get the binoculars for a closer look. She's afraid to put them to her eyes, I don't insist. *Crazy disease*. This woman spotted birds with these binoculars, now she's afraid of them.

"Rah, Rah, Rah," she calls, days later.

"Oh, Ca, they've hatched, you saw them. Thanks for showing me."

We watch parents feed their young, until one day she looks sad and calls, *"Rah, Rah."*

The babies have fallen from the nest and are on the cement surface. Later, we see them led by their mother to a bushy area where they will be safe.

I never thought I'd be thankful for such a small miracle.

By luck, or prayer, Marc calls. He's on his way to Ft. Lauderdale and thinking of moving to Florida. I'm happy for him but ask, "Can you come now, Marc? I need to go to the doctor and he may put me in the hospital." I've started hemorrhaging at times of the month thinking, *I can't get sick, there's no one to watch Carol.* He says, he will come as soon as possible.

Through the Alzheimer's support group, I get someone to stay with Carol while Marc takes me to the doctor. Thank God he corrects the problem at his office, and I return home with Marc. We talk after dinner, and he sees how Carol has declined. He's has a job interview and leaves after two days. I wonder if it's because he feels bad for his sister, or does he just want to get away from the sight of Carol pacing and gibbering to herself in the mirror—something new she's taken to do.

By the summer of '94, she paces until she falls from exhaustion. She lets me take her hand at times when I say, "C'mon Ca, let's lie down and get some rest." I lead her to bed, where she stays fifteen minutes, then is up pacing. She must have an alarm inside that says, 'keep going'.

She's forgotten how to sit so I take her to the couch, push down on her shoulders, and say, "Sit," as commanding an animal. Sometimes, she does if there's ice cream in front of her most of time she doesn't. When she does, I stroke her head and the back of her neck, give her chocolate ice cream while we watch *I Love Lucy* tapes. She taken to love funny movies and I try cartoons, but she doesn't like them, and leaves to pace. A movie of shooting, violence or loud noises, upsets her, and she yells at the television.

She's wetting the bed these and the pads I buy are too small, so I use a shower curtain. It covers where her body lays, works better than a pad; a hint from the support group.

Thank God for support groups. I buy an alarm, hang it on the front door, and lock the balcony doors at night afraid she'll climb over. I fear for her.

Her hearing is so sharp she hears the slightest noise; whereas, before the disease, she didn't. The rustle of sheets—she wakes, and is off pacing, no matter what hour.

I have someone stay with her while I attend the support group. I can't bring her anymore, it's impossible. I find help among these caregivers, like me. They are friends who laugh and cry with me.

Old friends want to hear only good stuff. They're not interested in the night she soiled the bed or how she shoved me out of the shower or yelled at the top of her lungs at someone in the mirror, herself.

At first, she liked the new friend in the mirror and grabbed my arm to show me. But I didn't understand, saying, "Ca, that's you, can't you see that?"

It's easier to go along with the new friend idea, it keeps her busy. She's happy talking to the new friend—*she* doesn't tell her what to do or when to eat.

When she wakes in the middle of the night, I lead her to the toilet so we won't have an accident. Soon as I leave, she's off the commode, pacing. I learn to sit on the bathroom floor and sing to her so she will stay. It's a new way of handling the disease, it works. So every two to three hours during the day, I lead her to the toilet and sing to her from the floor. Why won't she sit for any length of time? T*he doctors have no answers.* The group says, 'another stage'.

Sometimes I think back to when she went for that swim and didn't listen? I should have let her go. Maybe now, she'd be at peace.

After speaking with Dr. Ban, we decide to take her off all medication and let the disease take its course, as if it hasn't already? How did I think, *I* could make a difference?

13

During our year at the ocean, it was good to see the sunrise of a new day, even though it wouldn't be a perfect one. It was good to breathe the salt air and see fishermen in the morning. It was good to see a rainbow and make a wish for Carol's illness to be nonexistent. To watch a red moon come up over the ocean like a ball of fire, knowing all that God has made—but not understand why He wouldn't take away the disease.

We've moved back to Garden Parks. Our home has new walls, new carpet, bathroom tile—all fixed up. But for whom? There's only us, and we aren't much good for anything. I'm stressed and depressed, and Carol's gone into another world, walking away from this one.

Jay and Bea welcome us home and I wonder how I'm going to keep the place up. She paces all day, looking for an exit and once outside, the fear on her face is greater, because she's not where she thought she was. My guess is nothing looks familiar and she wants to go home. *Home*, to the place she knew as a child? When she smiles at pictures of her parents, and calls them by name. Does she think they're alive?

Her eating habits have changed. She uses her hands mostly, so I make finger foods. *She needs to keep her independence.* A bowl is easier; she scoops up food with a spoon, like soup, another piece of information from the group. Funny, the things that are important now. It used to be good golf shots, now it's if she'll use a spoon to eat.

I continue making vegetable juices of greens, beets, celery, carrots, and fruits so she gets nutrients. Her sugar craving astounds me. She looks in the fridge or cabinet for anything sweet.

She's afraid all the time, which I understand so well. She goes to her room, or tries to leave the condo when someone enters. She doesn't listen when I call her, so I keep cookies on hand at all times. She heads outside down the sidewalk and I run after her, "Ca, look what I have." Her eyes light up over a cookie. "C'mon Ca, follow me, and you can have the cookie." I feel I'm offering a bone to a dog instead of a cookie to my friend.

Thank God we have kind neighbors. Whenever they see her outside alone, they call me and I fly out after her.

When I'm on the toilet I leave the door open so I can hear her. If I hear the alarm, I jump up and run after her. Just like a two year old, except she's six-foot tall, with the strength of a horse. Her strength has gotten greater as the illness has progressed. Is it because the brain shuts down, and outer muscles become stronger; or is it because of the constant walking that she does?

When I lead her to the toilet, she puts on a face, as if it's a bad place to be. *What goes through her mind?* She no longer wipes herself. This is the hardest on me. She has accidents, and I strip her of clothing. When this first happened, I bought diapers for her to wear. One day she came to me with a look of worry.

"What's the matter?" I asked, as if I were going to get an answer. She looks toward her bathroom.

"What is it, Ca? Show me."

I followed her and saw water overflowing from the toilet. I shut off the underneath valve, cleaned up the mess, and was ready to call a plumber when I saw she was wet.

She let me undress her, and I found no diaper. I know where it is. Later the plumber found it.

I thought it was impossible for things to get worse, but they do. I hide sharp objects: scissors, letter openers, and any other items from her desk, because she's scratching furniture, and ripping up important papers. She pulls wallpaper off the bathroom wall, and I try a new tactic.

"Don't do that, Ca. You're hurting the wall."

It doesn't work, she gets angry, yelling in that other language. I decide, she can do whatever she wants, as long as she doesn't hurt herself.

I wonder if she's destroying everything that ever meant anything to her. She must be angry and frustrated over this illness, and not able to communicate it. The woman who graduated college, an English major, a brilliant person. *How? Why?*

This day I ask her while she paces, "Ca, can I see your necklace? I'd like to clean it."

She stops, looks at me and smiles, holds it up, making sounds, nodding her head.

I unhook the chain from her neck. She lets me, then I walk to the kitchen. She follows, watching me get the cleaner and cloth from the cabinet. I turn on the water faucet full force, and she turns her eyes toward it. I remove the small gold rose, slipping it in my pocket, and then remove her penicillin med alert and her mother's Virgin Mother charm. Her eyes back on what I'm doing she watches me clean. Her face happy seeing the shiny necklace. I put it on her. The gold rose, my first Christmas present to her some seven years ago, now she doesn't remember something we once shared. It hurts.

Out of a sound sleep, she jumps out of bed, yelling in that language I don't understand. I get out of bed, and try to calm her. I reach my hand out to her, "Please stop, Ca. C'mon, let's get a cookie."

She goes for me with the hairbrush she's picked up off the dresser. I move just in time. She hits the window blinds instead, then anything else that comes in her path. She sees something that I don't.

Into the dining room, she heads for the front door. She can't get out, I know. I've put a lock on high, near the upper frame. Again I try calming her, she swings and makes contact this time.

I run to my safe haven, and sit on the toilet seat lid. She's out there, yelling at the top of her lungs. She sees and hears someone I don't. She's on a rampage, hitting everything. I listen with the phone on my lap. *Should I call 911, have her committed?*

I hate watching her fade away into someone else. Calm once, a loving and understanding individual, she'd never hurt anyone or anything. Now she's an animal wanting to hurt everything. How did this happen? Why did it happen? For what reason? To teach me something? To teach her something? "God? If you hear me now, *please* calm her, make her 'normal', make her the loving person I once knew."

Will I keep my sanity? I'm sure she's lost hers. People have become afraid of her. *I've* become afraid of her.

I won't call 911. I'll go out there, somehow get pills in her. I'll give her, her favorite food, chocolate ice cream, open two capsules and blend the white powder in. She'll never know.

But when I go out there, things are bad, and I return to the bathroom. Roy comes to mind. He lives in the building next door. *I'll call him. He's big. He can handle her.*

Hoping she hasn't made her way to the kitchen where the knives are—all thoughts enter my mind. *She could hurt herself. She could hurt me.* Thank God for speed dial.

"Roy? It's Rose." I'm not waking him. I know, because he hasn't slept well since his wife died a few months ago.

"Carol's off the wall, yelling, and hitting everything in sight. Can you come over?"

"Sure, I'll be right there."

On days he goes for his morning walks to the ocean he stops by to say hello. I know I can depend on him, but now I need to unlock the door so he can get in. She's banging on it with the brush, the other hand pulling on the knob. She's even forgotten how to turn it. *There are good things.*

Can I get to the door and stay away from the brush? A loud knock startles her back into the dining room.

"Okay, I'm coming Roy," I yell, punching numbers disengaging the alarm. I slide back the bolt up top and open the door, see a friendly face. He can handle this insanity, the crazy person I'm living with.

Entering he calls her name, "Carol, hello."

She mutters something walking further into the living room.

"Oh, Roy, she's really lost it this morning. I need to get a pill in her fast and pray the neighbors haven't called the cops."

We wave our hands at her to come to the kitchen, she gibbers and waves back at us, to stay away.

I fill three bowls of cereal saying, "LET'S EAT BREAKFAST, ROY," hoping she'll hear, and come join us.

"OH, THIS IS REALLY GOOD, ISN'T IT?" I say, as I slip a spoonful of cereal in my mouth, then whisper, "*Is she coming?*"

"Yep, she's headed this way."

"HOW ABOUT SOME COFFEE, ROY?"

"That would be great!" he answers almost as loud. Hoping she'll be a part of us. *I know she must be hungry.*

She's at the doorway behind Roy, I see her. While pouring coffee, I put two sleeping pills in her cereal. "Hi Ca, how about something to eat?" putting her bowl on the table. "Come, sit here, next to Roy," and pull out a chair for her.

"Sha, Sha, Sha, Sha—Sha, Sha, Sha, Sha," she repeats. I hold the chair then push down on her shoulders, "Sit," I say, and she sits. I peel a banana and place it to the side of her bowl. We say nothing, she repeats, 'Sha'.

She picks up the banana and eats, me hoping she'll reach for the bowl with pills in it. I have no idea how this day will go unless she gets medication in her. Roy and I talk of weather, make believe she's not there. I've found, it's easier this way.

She's eaten half the banana and picks up the bowl. "Good Ca, eat it all," I say, but in less than five minutes she's finished, walking away with half a banana in her mouth.

"Thank God. Now she'll sleep. I don't know what I would have done without you, Roy. Thank you for coming." Tears come, tension released, fear gone.

He pats my head. "I'm glad I could help," he says. "You know you can call me anytime."

"I know. But I hate for anyone see her like this. You knew her when we swam in the pool. She wouldn't hurt a fly—now she's like an animal."

"Well, thanks for breakfast and remember, call me anytime," he says.

I hug and kiss him on the cheek, letting him out the door, and locking us in. I find Carol lying on her bed sleeping. I pull the throw over her. She's lost all sense of temperature and feel. She cut her finger awhile back before I put all sharp objects away. I saw blood on her shirt and asked, "What's this?" She shrugged. I spotted a cut on her thumb. She never felt it.

Covering her now, I lay next to her, staring at the ceiling. Thoughts of the kids and Ed come. *Is this the purpose? What path are 'You' trying to show me now?*

14

This morning, October 18, 1994, she's gotten the new rug and her pajamas soaked. She stood with legs apart and peed before I could take her to the bathroom.

"C'mon, Ca, time for a shower," I say.

It's a battle keeping her clean, not smelling of urine or other odors. One woman in the support group takes her husband outside in summer and washes him off with the garden hose. What I learn each day with the progression of this disease brings me back to when I was a child at times. Except then, we called them *hose fights*.

I undress her and coax her into the shower with me— another tip learned from the group. Fear is on her face but not the uncontrollable kind that I've come to know. I take the showerhead hose and spray myself.

"Oh—it feels *soooo* good. See, Ca. There's nothing to it." I sprinkle my feet then hers. "Doesn't the water feel nice?"

She steps back. I hope she's not going to be difficult today and reach for her hand as I did days ago. I spray her feet and legs, work up to her private areas, keeping the water away from her face. She slaps at me trying to push me. I used to wash her head at the kitchen sink when she could no longer go to the hairdresser. Those were easy days.

I've been putting off head washing for days now. Her hair is greasy. I know it needs to be washed today, before another week goes by. It's already three weeks. I spray her head, she pushes me hard against the glass doors. I give up.

"Okay, that's it. You're done." But before I get the words out of my mouth she's on a run through the living room, naked, wet, growling like a mad animal. How can this person be the one I knew so well?

Drying off, I want to spend the rest of the day here, in the bathroom. I want to fade into the walls and not be here or anywhere. I've lost her and nothing means anything. There are no dreams of future golf games to look forward to anymore.

Getting dressed, I pray she's calmed down. I grab towels, cookies, and head to her room. I find her talking to her friend in the mirror. She's calm. I understand why. The friend in the mirror isn't a threat. *I am.*

"Hey Ca, look what I've got."

She looks at the cookie—"*...Hmmm...*"—she's interested.

"Ca, come, sit on the bed," and I pat the towel I've laid out for her.

She comes, eyeing the cookie. I give it to her and press down on her shoulders. She sits and I dry her off as she munches.

"Good girl, you took a shower. You smell nice and clean now."

Putting on her blouse is easier these days. No bra anymore, that's impossible. I arrange a thick pad in her underwear and pull them up to her knees. Shorts are next, along with another cookie. I then pull *her* up and tug at her underwear and shorts till they're where they're suppose to be. She doesn't resist. She has her cookie.

Again I push down on her shoulders saying, "Sit." She does. *It's going well.*

Socks are next. I've learned to place one hand under her knee, another under her foot, then lift. She's forgotten how to raise her feet, except to pace. She lifts her knee to high, hitting my glasses into my eye. I yell, and run to the mirror to check. It stings, but my sight's okay. It's a fight to keep her clean, fed, and safe, everyday.

I return to her, eating a cookie. She's not aware she's even hurt me.

I try again. Her foot won't budge. It's glued to the floor.

"Please, Ca, lift your foot so I can put your socks and sneakers on."

Nothing.

Again I plead, "Please Ca, lift your foot."

Again, nothing.

"DO IT YOURSELF!" I yell, smacking her across the arm.

I run to *my* safe area—my bathroom.

"I can't keep this up. Please, Lord, help us. Please make it all go away."

A few minutes later I realize what I've done. I hit my friend—the person I loved and admired. It cuts through me like a knife.

In the kitchen, I get the phone book and dial.

"Good morning, Lacy Nursing Home," a woman answers.

"Hello, my name is Rose Lamatt. I need to place someone in your home," and feel a lump in my throat.

"Hang on, please. I'll get someone to help you."

Carol walks into the living room, cookies in hand, happy.

"Hello, Ms. Lamatt? This is Miss Randy. How can I help you?"

"I can't take it anymore! I just can't take it. I don't want to hurt her, but this morning was awful."

"Take a deep breath Ms. Lamatt, try to relax and tell me what's going on."

"I can't take it. I hit her this morning and that goes against everything I believe," I cry to a stranger. Spilling my guts to someone, I don't even know.

I tell this person all we've gone through, the helplessness, the loss. I have a connection, maybe she *can* help. Maybe she can save us from this disorder in life.

"Can you come in around three and bring Carol?"

"Yes. Thank you. We'll be there."

I hang up and see Carol looking out the sliding doors at birds in the backyard. A weight has been lifted off me. I'm relieved. It's for her. Hurting her is unforgivable.

"We'll get her later," Miss Randy tells me. "Let her walk through the halls. The aides will watch her."

Carol's gone off talking gibberish to others while I sign papers for her placement. In a fog, I know I need to do this now—otherwise I won't. Miss Randy is understanding, and tells me to bring her back tomorrow afternoon at one o'clock, with her personal items.

The ride home is quiet except for Carol's soft gibbering. At night, I give her sleeping pills and I lie awake. I should take one myself.

The next day I explain, "Ca, you're going on vacation for awhile to help others." She sits in the passenger seat, quiet, *possibly listening.* "You'll like it, Ca. The food's good and you can help people."

I feel she knows what's going on, or is it just my guilt kicking in. No, this will work. I can visit her everyday. She's only ten minutes away.

Miss Randy is waiting when we arrive. Carol walks past her down the hall. I try catching her. "She's all right. Let her go," the health care worker says.

I listen.

I stay three hours then I am told, 'Go home, get some rest, do something that's fun. We'll take care of her.'

I kiss her goodbye; she doesn't notice. She's busy with others and pacing.

Walking to the car, I feel free, yet alone, missing that someone by my side.

In the car I ask myself, "What do I do now? Do something that's fun?"

Where do I go for fun?

For years, she's all I've known, sick or not. I don't want to go home, it's empty. I call a neighbor, Fran, and tell her what's happened.

"Come, stay with me. I won't be home for awhile, the key's under the mat. Let yourself in."

At Fran's I let myself in and try to act normal when she comes home from work, but I can't, and go to *our* home and crawl into bed. I can't stand being without her and wrap my arms around her pillow, smell the scent of her hair on the fabric. I wish she were here, sick or not.

How could you leave me alone to face life? You were the sensible one, the smart one, the one who knew all the answers. How could you leave me? Why couldn't I be the sick one? Then I wouldn't have to face losing you. I cry, muffling the sounds so the neighbor on the other side of the wall won't hear.

Again—"God, where are You? I need You."

The next morning I shower, eat breakfast, dress, and head for the nursing home. I spot her walking fast through the hallways looking for a way out. *She's not aware I'm here*. I bring her to her room and change her clothes. They're the same ones I put on her yesterday. Under her fingernails are specks of feces. I smell it.

I stop an aide in the hall and ask how Carol was last night.

"She was up all night walking, but that's normal. It's better if you don't come often. That confuses her."

I try and understand. I guess it makes sense, and leave for home. It's empty. I don't hear her gibbering, see her pacing. It's quiet, lonely. I'm lost—like her.

Wednesday is the same. They tell me not to come. Thursday, I don't go, but call. They say she's fine and not to worry. I feel better that I've spoke to someone, envision her in activities or eating with professionals handling the disease.

Friday I meet her at the front door trying to get out. She looks awful, bruises and a black eye. I take her hand, "Come with me, Ca." She doesn't resist.

I ask an aide, "What happened to her? Did she fall?"

No answer. I realize she may not speak English. I ask the nurse the same question—no answer either.

On our way to her room, I watch her stumble. She looks drunk, like someone living on the streets.

Along the wall near the bathroom we pass a dirty diaper lying on the floor. She reaches for it.

"No, Ca. Leave it there." The feces under her nails.

I wash her face, comb her hair, she tries brushing her teeth. We make our way to the dining room for lunch. I pass an aide, and tell her of the dirty diaper.

For lunch she has a bologna sandwich, milk, and banana, devours everything. *Has she eaten?* Later, sitting on the porch she bobs her head, wanting sleep. I stroke the back of her head, then lead her to her room for a nap. She lays down, and I stroke her arm.

I study my friend sleeping. She's exhausted from her new surroundings. They haven't watched her the way I thought they would. I had thought, the more people the better. But they don't love her the way I do. She doesn't mean anything to them. It's just a job. Bruises on her arms, face and hands, and a black eye tells me so. I pray, *Dear Lord, what am I supposed to do? I'm so tired. You know, she's all I have.*

She's caged, treated badly, and no one understands her, except me. *What have I done?—I'm the one who put her here!*

While she naps, I walk the hall. I hear a woman call, "I need to go to the bathroom!"

How wonderful she can speak and tell them what her needs are. But no one comes to her rescue.

I go to the nurses' desk. "The woman in 109 needs to go to the bathroom," I tell the nurse.

"Someone will help her," she replies.

Half an hour goes by. Now the woman is crying.

When Carol wakes, I lead her to the bathroom, where the dirty diaper still lays. I wash her face, comb her hair, and set her on the toilet. She doesn't fight me.

I mention the dirty diaper to a new nurse at the desk, and ask her to call the doctor for me. I'd like to speak with him. She says she will. I thank her and bring Carol into the activity room hoping others will be there. Many are sitting in wheelchairs, sleeping or doing nothing. I notice the same-drugged look as Carol's on *their* faces. I turn on the radio and we sit and listen to music.

Later at dinner, Carol has a bowl of chicken soup in front of her, but is more interested in the woman sitting across from her, without food. She pushes her bowl to the woman, nodding for her to eat.

"No, Ca. The lady will get her food in a minute," and I slide the bowl back to Carol. Nothing comes from the kitchen for the woman.

I hate this place.

The woman finally gets her dinner, as Carol finishes hers. I take her back to her room and pass the dirty diaper on the floor. She tries picking it up, I stop her. I wonder why she's easier to handle here than at home? *Medications?* I watch her brush her teeth, and feel heat from within me rise to anger. I see her face in the mirror, that beautiful human being that I'd come to know so well.

Throwing her clothes in a garbage bag, I tell her, "Come on Ca, we're going home."

I take her hand and walk to the nurses' station.

"I'm taking Carol home."

"For the evening?"

"No. She's not coming back."

"You can't do that."

"Watch me. No ones looked after her. Just look at the bruises she has," and point to her arm and eye. "No one's given me any answers to what's happened to her. We're going home."

I lead her to the car, throw the plastic bag in the back seat, and help her sit down. She doesn't fight me. We head for home. I'm calmer knowing she's with me and won't get hurt. As we near our condo she smiles and points. *She recognizes where she is.*

Inside, I fix milk and cookies and we sit on the sofa watching *I Love Lucy* tapes. My arm around her shoulder, like always, she doesn't get up. She falls asleep and I sit content feeling her presence. After a while I wake her, and lead her to bed. Again she doesn't resist. *She must have gone through hell.*

I lay with her, stroking her arm, as tears run like tiny rivers. She falls into a deep sleep, jerky movements as she's done for a long time.

Later in the living room alone, I recap what's happened this past week. Someone from 1985 comes to mind and I make the call.

15

Hi Jan? It's Rose."

"Well, hello there! Where have you two been? All we get are Christmas cards from you. Is everything okay?"

"Oh Jan, it's a long story."

How could I forget one of our first neighbors in Florida? The great cook, who served us wonderful dinners, then afterward we'd play word games or charades, then she'd leave for her night job, a nurse. I cry, giving her the short version of what's been happening, then the recent one, *todays*.

"Lacy Nursing Home?—that's the worst! Where is she now?"

"She's sleeping. They drugged her so bad she's like a zombie."

"You can't keep her home, Rose."

"Yes, I know. I'd love to, but I can't. She's six feet tall you remember, and has lost her speech. She's stronger than an ox and yells in a language I don't understand. I know the neighbors have had it."

"You sound awful. I know what you're talking about, I work for Wheitz Nursing Home and see it all day long. Let me talk with the administrator. I'll let him know Carol's my friend and needs help now. Suppose I get back to you Monday?"

"God, Jan—I don't know if I can wait that long. If I don't do it now, I never will."

"Listen, with the drugs she has in her, she'll probably sleep tonight and tomorrow. Do you have anything to sedate her if needed?"

"Yeah, she's been on all kinds of medication: antianxiety, antidepressant, sleeping pills. You name it...she's been on it."

"If she gets impossible, give her sleeping pills to keep her down. I'll call you Monday morning." I thank Jan and hang up.

Maybe it's a good idea to put her where Jan works. She could watch her everyday, and let me know what's happening. There's only one negative. It's forty-five minutes away.

I get into bed, Carol on my left. It's nice to have her home. I lay awake a long time. She sleeps through the night and most of the next day. Sunday she's up little and easy to care for.

Monday Jan calls at nine-thirty, as promised. "Hi Rose. How'd it go over the weekend?"

"Pretty good. She slept mostly."

"I'm in the admissions office. Ann, head of admissions, would like to speak with you."

"Okay."

"Hello, Mrs. Lamatt?"

"Yes."

"Jan has filled me in on you and Carol. If you agree, I'll ask Lacy Nursing Home to fax over Carol's records and you can bring her in tomorrow morning around nine. Jan thinks very highly of you both, and that's enough for me."

"Thank you for helping on such short notice. I have copies of all Carol's records, so I'll bring them with me."

"As I said, Jan has told me all I need. I look forward to meeting you both."

I thank her again, knowing I must do this. If I don't, I'll be dead before her, then who will care for her? Slapping her, was not acting in *her* best interest.

I call Izzy and Kim, support group comrades. They say they'll go with me tomorrow. I feel better.

For Carol's last day home, I want to spend every moment with her, even if I have to follow her pacing. Funny though, she doesn't pace today.

I try coaxing her outside for a walk around the complex; she balks, wanting inside only. Her interest is chocolate chip cookies. So we sit watching TV, eating cookies. At times I look at her face, thinking how much I've come to know it. Tears come, knowing soon it will be gone.

Getting her to bed is easy. I ask if she wants apple juice, and she smiles. I wonder, does she know what's ahead? Calm, relaxed the whole weekend— why couldn't she be like that all the time? Then I wouldn't have to let her go.

Opening a capsule, I sprinkle the powder in a glass of juice and stir, remembering when she'd spit the pills back at me until I learned to fool her. I felt I was deceiving her then. Now I know she needs it, God knows what will happen; yelling, throwing things, who knows? The neighbors sure are tired. They kept telling me I had to do something or I was going to have a stroke. They loved her too, and hated to see the person she'd become.

In bed I sleep little, wanting to be awake for her last night. I touch her arm at times feeling her there, and listen to her snore. Soon things *will* be different.

I lay there remembering Carol of the past:

Carol is a loving person to everyone and every creature she meets. A woman in front of us in line at the grocery store doesn't have enough money to pay her bill. Carol reaches in her pocketbook and hands the clerk money. The woman nods her thanks, but I see more than that. I see a love passed on.

Walking to a restaurant for breakfast after golf, we see a young woman covered in filth. When seated, the young woman comes in and sits across from us. The waitress asks her to leave. Carol calls the waitress over and tells her to give the woman anything she wants, put it on our bill. When finished eating, we get up to leave, the young woman is eating eggs and pancakes, she nods her thanks. Again, I see the love passed on.

Carol sends money to friends, who are in need for their children's college expenses. She buys a tool for a young golf pro who has opened his own business. She takes young golf pros to the exclusive golf club she belongs to and pays their fees. They are in awe to have played a course they could never have played without her gift.

I see anyone who comes in contact with her loves her. She thinks of the other person, always. She cares for injured birds, animals of any kind. She doesn't even kill the tiny lizard that has entered our home. She picks it up with a paper towel, brings it outside, and tells me, 'We are all connected in some way.'

This Tuesday, Izzy and Kim sit in their cars waiting. I toss Carol's suitcase in the trunk and think of the appointment in West Palm Beach, not a happy one.

After fastening her seat belt I press down the lock and close the door. Izzy and Kim sit in the back seat.

Carol makes noises in her voice. *We* talk of weather and news.

Once there, I offer a cookie, pulling on her to get her out of the car. I hold her hand walking to admissions. My heart beats fast, skips. No matter—I wish I *would* die.

Ann meets us, "I see you made it down all right?"

"Yes, the drive wasn't bad." I lie. It was for me.

"I'm happy to meet you in person, Rose"—Ann extends her hand, the way Carol used to.

"These are friends, Kim and Izzy. They're my support this morning."

"Nice to meet you both."

"And this is Carol." I bring the hand I'm holding to Ann, but Carol brings it down.

Ann touches her shoulder, "Hello, Carol, it's nice to meet you."

She doesn't respond. *Does she know?*

Ann offers her a seat, but Carol's one with my hand. Ann asks her questions, then looks at me, "Doesn't she speak?"

"No, not our language," I smile.

Minutes later, her agitation starts. I nod to Izzy.

"Ca, go for a walk with Izzy."

"Yes, c'mon Carol, let's go find some pretty flowers." And she goes with Izzy, offering the cookie.

Kim takes a seat in the hall. Now it's business, me and Ann. I know this part already. I did it last week.

"I received information from Lacy Nursing Home," Ann says. "What papers do you have with you?"

"Everything from day one. All her medical records."

Ann looks at papers, Carol's medical briefcase I've added to over the years. "Good she's had a chest x-ray—we won't need to repeat it. I'll make copies," and calls her secretary.

She hands me a packet about the Home to keep, and tells me to sign where the check marks are. I sign my name and print Carol's in red. I feel I'm signing a life away. In a sense, I am—two.

Jan comes in and hugs me.

"Oh Rose, I'm so sorry. I just saw Carol outside. She's changed so much. I can't believe it."

I hold back tears. I haven't seen Jan in four years. She's put on weight, like me. She'd known us when we were happy, healthy, eating dinners she'd prepared, playing card games.

I call Carol and Izzy inside, and Ann escorts us to the second floor, to Carol's room. I hold her hand leading her, even though she wants to lead me elsewhere.

"Let her go," Ann says. "She can't get outside. The aides will keep an eye on her."

Ann has made it known the ratio of patients to aides is seven to one. Versus, Lacy's ten to one. I let her go. It's rating in nursing home magazine is high, if that means anything. Lacy's is also.

I check her room while Izzy and Kim place themselves on couches near the elevators.

It's a nice room. Private. It smells clean, pretty, blue drapes, *her favorite color*, white bed spread with bed rails, a blue recliner, dresser desk combo with TV. What bothers me? The forty-five minute drive. *Jan will watch her.* I put her clothes in the closet and leave. Someone's playing the piano in the activity room, where I find Izzy, Kim and Carol.

"Rose, it might be better if you left while she's busy," Ann says.

Reluctantly, I tell the others, 'we better go'. Funny even Lacy Nursing Home wanted you out, makes you feel you're not needed, a leftover, kicked out. Again I'm told not to visit, this time for a month.

I walk toward the elevator turn around and watch her in the activity room, trying to make contact with other residents. She seems happy, even though no one understands her. Getting in the elevator, the doors close, and I lose sight of her. She's on her own now. So am I.

Later in bed, I cry knowing my fear of driving will keep me from seeing her face. I know it's for good this time. She's not coming back. I sleep, waking often. *Is she walking the halls looking for me? Is she falling, or is she, perhaps, sleeping?*

16

Don't visit until she learns who's caring for her. She has to learn a new environment." I listen but want say, 'research shows Alzheimer victims can't learn *anything* new, so how can she learn a new environment?'

I'm lost without her. Past Thanksgivings were full of love, my family, and our friends. I remember the first one; our arrival in Florida, we played golf. I remember and remember, and want to forget, like her.

No one can care for her the way I did, *no one*. Know her every move, what she wanted, what she didn't. Jan assures me on our weekly phone calls, 'She's fine Rose, take care of yourself'. Thank God she's on the second floor and can't get into the streets, like the woman I read about in the newspaper last week, found a day later in the woods.

Christmas I have strength for the drive, my relaxation is tape playing. We'll have dinner together, instead of me staying home.

At the four-story building, I walk past the admissions office where I stood not that long ago. I press number two in the elevator, and see my first sight of her, pacing. W*hat* *else did I expect—her sitting watching television?* I put my arm around her shoulder.

"Merry Christmas, Ca."

She smiles speaking words I still don't understand.

"Are you ready for Christmas dinner?" I ask.

An aide looks at me as if I'm crazy.

I seat her, she gets up. I seat her, she gets up. This goes on until I finally give up, and let her pace down two hallways. I then take her hand, and lead her outside to the screened balcony. "Look at the pretty plants," hold a flower to her. "Ca, look at the color. Isn't it beautiful?"

No answer. I understand.

Next to a chair I place my hands on her shoulders and set her down, then sing, "Oh, we ain't got a barrel of money," she laughs. Soon she's up, through the door, long strides move down one hall.

Catching up, I grab her hand, "C'mon Ca, let's get some chocalotta ice cream." She stops, stares at me with those big brown eyes. I can't believe she still knows the word.

We pass the nurses' station, and I tell an aide we're going downstairs for ice cream. She nods. I push the elevator button. Doors open, and Carol runs inside the small box, alarm blaring at the bracelet on her wrist. I disengage the noise and hit number one. She gibbers for the short ride. The doors open, and her legs go into action pulling me behind her.

At the ice cream parlor, I meet Valerie, the attendant, and ask for one chocolate ice cream, telling her what Carol called it.

"I've never heard that before, it's cute," and hands me one bowl of chocalotta with a spoon.

I head outside, her hand in mine. Seating her, I get a chair for myself.

"So tell me, how are you doing?" giving her the ice cream.

She eats, as if it's the last ice cream on earth.

"Are they taking good care of you, my friend? Are you sleeping nights? Do they sing to you the way I do?" My questions go unanswered, but that's okay.

In minutes, she drops the empty Styrofoam bowl on the ground, up to pace.

I throw the bowl away and grab her hand. "Let's go for a walk around the pond." I see that look—the happy one.

Maybe this is the right place for her.

Walking, we see turtles and ducks; she gibbers to them, and then looks at me. I smile. Seeing cars on the road, she looks fearful as they whoosh by.

"Yes, they're going fast, aren't they?"

Her eyes wide "It's okay, Ca. There's nothing to be afraid of," reassuring her, I hope.

We've gotten a workout, three laps around the pond. She's on drugs to keep her calm, not like others that made her stumble and fall. They're trying new med's to see what works best.

Back in her room I surf the television, finding golf. *She might take an interest*, but it's short-lived, she's up to pace. I watch her awhile, then decide to leave. I don't say goodbye. I don't want to disrupt her pacing. I tell the nurse to take good care of her. She tells me, she will.

106

Inside the elevator, I push the button and take my last sight of her. "God bless you, Ca." She doesn't look my way or see where I've gone. She's in a world all her own. An imagine of a caged animal comes to mind, saddening me. The doors close.

Walking to the car, tears pool—it hurts to leave her. Nothing I've ever done has hurt this much. I don't want to live, watching her like this.

Finding another world, like her, I take myself to the movies. It takes time, but finally I'm in a fantasy world, seated eating popcorn and drinking soda, with others around me. They laugh at the screen. *I try.*

17

The fear is with me all the time. My feet are stuck in wet cement. I can't go anywhere, do anything, just like the sixteen year old; fast heart beats, dizzy, sweats—everything's the same. In bed, I pull the covers over my head—as if that will help? It didn't years ago. People say they care, but that doesn't matter, because I don't matter to myself. I feel I'm living outside my body, watching from a distance—encapsulated in a bubble where nothing gets through, to make me feel.

I struggle not knowing who the real person is. Am I the caregiver? Am I the child of my mother and father or the wife of my husband? Am I the mother of my children? Or the person full of fear that I know so well? Am I the unforgiving person, the loving person, the child of God? Or am I all the above?

I hate these thoughts of insecurity—that come often whether waking disoriented from a "sleeping dream", or in an "awake-in-life" dream, as today. Why can't I find the answer?

Will the real you please stand up?

If God knows the 'real' me, why am I not shown her? Why do I go through these self-crucifixions that scar deeply every time they hit? I'm dead inside, have lost my soul—this must be the answer. "Please, God, answer me, comfort me, let me rest in Your Love."

It's January '95, I want to rid the condo of everything that has anything to do with Carol. *How could she leave me?*

Her lawyer says, I can keep the condo until her money runs out, then I'll need to sell it. If we were married, I'd be able to keep the condo and the car. We're not. According to Florida law even though she cannot care for herself, she can keep the condo and car. *Is she ever coming back to this place? No. Is she ever going to drive again? No.* The love I have for her will just go on forever. Go figure laws. Mad, lonely, hurt, I feel displaced.

It's costing $4,000 a month for her room and $4,000 for private-duty-aides, because the regular nursing home aides can't handle her six-foot body. It takes everything a person owns to pay for this disease, sucking up all one's assets, then the person goes on Medicaid. It makes no sense. I won't have her in a 'county home', where homeless people go. That's for people who don't have anyone who cares about them. I want the best care for her. I need to sell the condo.

I give the listing to Fran, neighbor and realtor. When strangers come to look at our home I'm embarrassed, angry, and furious at what they say, "Oh, it needs this," and "We have to change the colors," and on and on.

It's a beautiful home, once filled with love and laughter. It has beautiful memories—why can't they see that? This is the place I didn't want to move to because of those vague feelings I had. I know now why—Carol's illness. But we'd made it into a home despite that feeling, and now people say they want to change it. I go for walks when the lookers come. I wonder where I'll move to? I have no idea. I'm taking each day as it comes, and they're all bad. Sometimes I feel like an ant, running around in circles, going nowhere.

Within the month, an older couple decides to buy it.

The complex has a group of men and women, that do yard work, clean clubhouses and pools. I ask one if he will help me with heavy items and decide to give him the furniture, except the dining table we loved. We'd spent weeks shopping for just the right table and color. I decide to give it to Carol's favorite charity, one that comforts people in the last stages of life.

I leave her bedroom as is, and make the guest room home base. It has a small television I can watch in bed. The kitchen table is small with two chairs. I'll keep those. I rid the condo of things I won't use and rent a storage unit keeping items we shared: my mother's lamp, pictures, sheets and towels, just in case I ever find a way to live again. I keep her clothes for the nursing home, which seem to be leaving faster than I can bring them to her. I know I'm being lied to when the staff says her clothes were lost in the laundry. There's no way for me to prove stealing. I've thought of a camera in her room, just to see. But, what's the use? If they need clothes that badly, let them have them.

I save her bedroom for last. Her paperwork, personal items, clothing, perfumes I smelled on her, shoes, photo albums of golf—items playing golf with me. All of it needs to go.

She has two closets: one for everyday clothes, another for dressy clothes, parties, dinners out. She loved shoes and handbags, carries one with her now. *Maybe she thinks she's going somewhere?* The support group tossed this thought around. 'The restlessness of the illness makes them prepared to go somewhere—possibly back to their home of long ago?'

"God, I wish I understood this disease," picking up a handbag, I throw it in a garbage bag.

I work at a panic pace filling large garbage bags, putting them outside in the dumpster. I want everything gone, out of my sight.

So many memories to go through—so much of her — pictures, her mother, father, Anne, golf albums…so much one person could keep. *I guess this is what a person's all about: what they collect over a lifetime. Now, she knows none of it.*

In the hall closet on the top shelf are boxes, one marked *Christmas.* What do I do with this? And think of the holidays we shared, the first Charlie Brown tree. Wh*at do I do with the ornaments now?*

I write storage on it.

I sit at her desk—where she spent much of her time, writing friends, family, and congressmen on snags in our country.

'Write a letter,' she'd say, when I told her how disgruntled I'd become over our country's issues. I thought of the many times I'd called her to dinner, and she'd say, 'Okay, just one more line to write.'

I go through her personal papers, run across a folder marked, *Rose.* A vivid scene in her condo up north comes to mind. 'Rose, if you need money, it's in this envelope,' she'd said.

How embarrassed I was then. Now opening the envelope, I see the same $300. I don't want this. I want you. I want your laughter, our golf games. I don't want this money!

Anger over a rotten illness bubbles inside me, tears ask to come and I let them. I quit, lay down awhile. I'm still an hour, then think I need to get this done, *get up.*

In the back of her desk drawer I run across her little black daily entry books, like the one she'd scribbled my name in for our first golf date. I thumb through pages, toss them to the black garbage bag on the floor. I watch, hear them hit the bag, then think, *should I keep them*? Picking them up, I put them in a bag marked *Storage.* I find greeting cards I'd given her—cards of congratulations on winning tournaments—throw them in the garbage bag.

I finally close her bedroom door. The room is done. Boxes and bags labeled, what to keep, what to throw out, and what goes to storage for a later date.

Almost a month later, I still don't know where I'm going. My visits to her are few and short. Fear keeps me from taking the long drive.

The closing date for the condo is set. Years ago, I didn't want to live in this place because of a premonition. Now I don't want to leave. A thought lifts my heart.

The closing takes an hour. I'm handed a check for a large sum of money and deposit it in her trust account. I tell the person handling it to make sure the nursing home gets paid if anything happens to me.

Back home, I collect my belongings, two suitcases. I check rooms, closets, making sure everything's gone and leave the keys on the kitchen counter along with a note. '*I hope you'll be as happy as I was here*'.

At the front door, I turn for one last look, a flash of love and happiness come, and a vision of Carol's laughing face.

I close the door.

18

May 1995 the guard gate lifts as it did in, '84 and '93, when my dear friend was with me. Funny, how I always felt God was here maybe because of the calm I felt. Back to where it all began. I park in the underground garage and wait for the elevator. Doors open, glass mirrors. Ten years since that night of blue blazer reflections, when we were on our way out to dinner. *Who would think two lives could change so much over such a short period?*

Unlocking the door, I drop my bags and head to the balcony. Clean, fresh salt air fills my lungs. How much easier it is to breath here. I sit a minute, then look to see if the doves are building a nest, nothing. People are in the pool, the ocean's rough, as a nor'easter has blown in. There are whitecaps as far as the eye can see, and windsurfers getting their fun for the day.

Back inside I hang my clothes in the master bedroom closet—*Carol's*. Going through the linen closet, I pull sheets and towels out to wash, throwing them on the floor. I have no idea who's been here since we left a year ago. I find a rolled-up golf sock tucked in the back, a blue dot on the toe. Carol's—her dot was blue, mine purple, so we could tell them apart when washed. I stare at it. "You son of a gun, you hid it here for me. You know how I hate to be alone. Thanks, Ca."

I tape the saying she gave me so many years ago behind the medicine cabinet door: *Don't look forward, the everlasting Father looks after you...* and read it, wondering now, How can you not look forward?

After straightening, I drive around the corner to the grocery store. It's good to be home.

It's been awhile since I've done anything but care for her, now I find the days simple. I go to the Alzheimer's support group once a week, looking forward to visiting with old friends of four years. Using the Internet, I search for information on Alzheimer's to bring them. There's a bond among us that others can't possibly relate to. The group lives each other's fears and happiness when we talk of our week's events. Lucky for me, we meet around the corner from where I live. I visit my friend once a week, even though driving the distance makes me panic.

Marc calls saying John has passed away, and sadness fills me. Almost a year now since Mom's left. I guess he couldn't live without her. *Can I go on without Carol?* I'll remember John for the happiness he brought. When he came into the house and played the piano love flowed from where it usually wasn't. God bless John.

Late one afternoon, I feel Carol calling. Trying not to dwell on this I do paperwork. But the call gets stronger. *'I need you—come!'*

I dress, in a haze. *I have to go.* I told her I'd never abandon her. Fear is with me, but not strong enough. *"I'm coming, Ca,"* leaving the garage.

In the car the radio plays loud music blocking out fear. It comes, but her call overshadows it.

Once there, I'm better. Passing the nurses' station, I say hello, and continue to the last room on the left. *Door closed, Why?* It's usually open unless they're dressing her or she's sleeping, but even then, it's left slightly ajar. I hear the television, *normal*. Her private aide leaves it on while Carol naps.

Opening it slowly, thinking she's napping, I see her private aide lying on the bed watching television and an aide from the floor sitting in a chair. Both laughing. I see Carol to the left of me in the bathroom, banging her fist on the mirror.

"What the hell do you think you're doing!" I yell.

"You see this woman"—pointing to Carol, "she's paying you to watch *her*, not the TV!" One aide hurries past me out the door.

"Dammit," I yell to the private aide. "I'm paying you to make sure she doesn't get hurt. Do you even care what happens to her? DO YOU?"

She doesn't respond. Carol stops banging, and looks at me. The aide walks toward Carol.

"Don't touch her. Get out. You're fired," my hand outstretched toward the exit.

"You can't do that."

"Oh, yes I can! Get out!"

Carol's eyes are wide, nodding her head, almost saying, '*You're right. I'm glad you came.*'

Donna, the director of nurses comes.

"Mrs. Lamatt, can we please go to my office?"

"No," then pointing to the aide. "I don't want that woman near Carol. As far as I'm concerned, she's gone."

"Calm down, Mrs. Lamatt. Come with me where we can discuss this."

"I don't need to discuss it. Did the aide tell you what happened? Did she tell you, she and the floor aide were watching television, not Carol?"

Donna turns to the aide, and gets no response.

"I'm sorry Donna, but this is very upsetting. I'm going to bring it to the administrator's attention. It shouldn't have happened. This woman"—nodding toward Carol—"is paying a lot of money to be kept safe. If she didn't need it, she wouldn't be here."

"I'm sorry. I didn't know the whole story." Donna tells the aide to leave and it will be reported. I have her word.

I thank her, saying, "I'd like some time with my friend, now."

Combing Carol's hair I tell her how pretty she looks, seeing our reflections in the mirror. We're calm now.

We make our way to the ice cream parlor, then outside. At the end of my visit, I stop at the office where aides are hired.

I don't understand why people can't do their job. Why would television be more important than their patients? *Why do these workers stay in health care?*

The drive home is easier.

As time goes by, I push myself to leave the condo, otherwise it's the same as when I was married, homebound. I drive around the neighborhood hearing sounds, seeing things, but nothing registers. I stop at a store, carry on a conversation with the clerk. It brings me back to reality. I drive through the car wash, listen to the brushing sounds, watch the monster strips cover the car, as if it were seaweed under the ocean. I think of the times Hope and I went through a wash just like this. We'd pretend we *were* under the ocean. 'Here comes an octopus,' I'd say and she'd scream. It brings me back into the real world, except Hope isn't around anymore. Matthew either.

Two things are saving me, the sun coming up over the ocean each morning, and the sight of people below in the pool having fun. It keeps me from feeling alone.

Why would someone who brought the good out in me, be taken from me?

911 is dialed in the middle of the night. Anxiety attack, they say, caused my irregular heartbeats, they offer me tranquilizers. I'm reliving old years. Ed's fighting me every inch of the way on divorce, and I don't care anymore. My lawyer tells me I need to be in New York, but I can't go anywhere, except stay in the little world I know. Everything's coming down on me—fears, Carol, no divorce, soon, no money.

Why don't you take the elevator—you've been thinking about it for months. Go ahead, you're feeling strong today.

Dressed in blue shorts, yellow golf shirt, and Carol's V-neck sweater wrapped around my shoulders, I walk the catwalk. I have one thought; my mind not cluttered. I push the button, watch lights, G—ground floor, garage—three, doors open. I step inside; notice mirrors, seeing a blur of blue/yellow with a V-neck. My fingers brush over the buttons...I push fourteen.   No   thoughts,   just numbers...five, six, ten —Debbi's floor...a blur, fourteen, doors open.

I move forward—as I did playing golf—on a mission. Once out of the elevator I turn right, ocean side, red lighthouse in the distance. Everything small, tiny, minuscule, nothingness, like me. People in the pool look like ants. *I've been here before, Hope and Carol wanted to take pictures. Fun then. I must stop thinking of the past and go forward.*

A strong wind blows, and out at sea a mist connects to the horizon. The sun is in the afternoon sky making shadows over sand and pool. *All I need to do is climb over the four-foot rail...do I have the guts?*

"NO!—stop thinking or you won't!"

Dry mouth, heart pounding. Not important. Hands on cold, hard railing, I lean over, making my head swirl. *Remember the first time you were dizzy looking down?* Stop thinking!

Blue/green ocean where God was. Ha, where are You now? All my life I've believed in You. How could I ever trust You with my Journey?

I've waited too long, thoughts are speeding in. What are you doing? He *is* here...He really *is*. You can't do this—it wouldn't fulfill His plan. He can make everything right—have faith. *Where did that come from? Not me.*

My heart settles. A new look comes. *Yes, it is beautiful, but there's more here than the eye can see.* I see the beauty. I heard the *Voice.* It wasn't my voice. My thoughts are only negative ones. I have another chance to change my way of thinking.

Friday afternoon my lawyer calls, saying I need to be in court Monday, for 'the divorce hearing', otherwise, the judge is throwing the case out. After all these years, it's getting thrown out? Ten years of Ed's 'no billable hours'.

My thoughts go to him. 'Son of a bitch, all those years while you got your degrees, I stayed home changing diapers, cooking. You open your business, it does well, and this is how you repay me? *You* know what I went through living with you—you know the panic attacks, the fears. You're doing it purposely to keep *your* house, *your* car, and everything else that you said was yours. All I ever was, was chief cook and bottle washer, while you went out for your three-hour martini lunches with so-called 'clients'. Did you think I was *that* stupid? Why did you have this hatred for me—because I left you? But, we had agreed: you knew it was a bad marriage from the beginning. Did you want me living on the streets, pushing a cart with whatever belongings I had left? Most of the time, I treated you with kindness even when you drank your water glasses full of vodka. Every night, I had dinner on the table when you walked in the door. I washed your clothes, pressed and folded them. In the beginning, you asked me, 'should I go into business?' I told you, "Yes, do it now; otherwise, you never will. I have faith in you. You can make it work." I bet you turned the kids against me. I guess this is the way you repay me.

I lay in bed later unable to sleep, feeling nothing but hatred for the man I'd married. Exhausted I gave my thoughts over to God, and fell into a deep sleep. I woke in the middle of the night going straight to the computer, typing a letter, "Dear Judge: Neither you nor Ed can take anything from me, because what I have no one can take. It is a gift from God. I have *Me*. If you want to leave me without money, that's fine, because God is the only one who can take anything from me."

Three pages of words came from somewhere above me, then out my fingers. Somehow, I knew God wasn't going to take from me, because if anything, He'd given me life back. The next day I sent the letter, overnight, return receipt requested. On Monday late afternoon, the lawyer called saying the judge had read my letter in court, which he seldom did. As a result, the decision went slightly in my favor. I would get alimony every month, plus a yearly distribution. No one could take from me ever again.

19

Almost a year has passed since I moved here, seven months after my fourteenth-floor endeavor. I'm in the pool exercising, riding my bike and walking the ocean searching for shells. It's nice to be among the living.

I meet Debbi at the pool and go over my thoughts, good ones, and bad ones. She's become a friend, counselor with weekly visits. I remember the first day I met her at the tar station in '93 with Carol. She's stood by me through fear and Alzheimer's. I know at times I'm not a good patient, sometimes falling back into my old habits. But I'm trying.

I'm writing about Carol and life with her, but at times I get upset, and put it away in a drawer.

This day, in July of '96, I find Carol in bed with a urinary tract infection. I see her body flat to the mattress with only her head showing, she's lost so much weight. The aide has the television on.

"How she doing, Mavis?"

"Oh, she's a little under the weather today. The antibiotics are making her sleep a lot."

I tell Mavis to get lost for awhile, that I'll feed Carol lunch. She thanks me and leaves. I remember when I didn't get along with Mavis. I yelled a lot back then. She took it, and now she helps Carol just by being close to her. This was all I ever wanted from them—to be near so she wouldn't get hurt, see that she's fed and diapers changed. This was all I ever wanted.

She sleeps. I pull a chair close, take hold of her hand. She looks so peaceful, quiet. Is this the same person who threw me out of the shower? *Why couldn't you be like this at home? Then I wouldn't have had to put you here.* Other patients are quiet, easygoing, but not you. You were the strong one—always.

I look deep into her face, words come, "I want nothing more than for you to be well, but that doesn't seem to be happening. I'm praying you will pass from this life. It's heartbreaking to see you like this. I can't see the purity in you today. Why? I feel we're not connected."

I turn away so tears won't come, but they do. Will I ever get used to *this* Carol? If I can't see the purity in her, it's not in me either.

Oh Ca, how I wish you could hear my cries.

Leaning over, I look for the love in her. I cry the whole time, trying to put my energy into her. "I'm so sorry, Ca. You, of all people, didn't deserve this. No one does. Why does this happen to good people?"

Oh, Ca. I love you and hate seeing you like this. The aide tells me you're up nights walking the floors. I wonder if you are looking for me. That idea makes me sad, and I hope you're just getting exercise that you always loved.

She doesn't open her eyes. I tickle her trying to wake her. Her eyes stay shut. The aide returns, we get her out of bed, she can't do it on her own anymore. We take her to the toilet, and I kneel on the floor and sing to her. She's doesn't know to look up.

After I feed her, she falls asleep. I leave. I cry on my drive back to the ocean, finding comfort in bed.

My lease at the ocean is up. I love it so, and don't want to leave this place I've come to call home. I've grown here, learning of me. I decide to stay another six months, until my savings run out. A gift from Mom. I know she would approve.

"Carol's fallen," The nurse says on her phone call.

"Is she all right?" I ask.

"Yes. She had x-rays. Nothing's broken."

"Give her a kiss for me," I say and hang up.

How could she fall? She has round-the-clock aides. Maybe they're not watching her. Maybe they're watching television again?

The next day, I look for her roaming the hall, she isn't. I find her in her room sitting watching television with an aide—a new one.

"Hi. Why is she sitting?" I ask the aide.

"Hi Ca, how're doing?" bending to kiss her and introduce myself to the aide. Her tag reads, Cathy.

"Good to meet you, Cathy. How come she's not up running around?"

"I think something's wrong."

"What do you mean?"

"I've been here since seven, and every time she gets up, she moans and sits back down. I told the nurse at the desk. She thinks Carol bruised herself falling."

"Oh, maybe." Kneeling, I look at her. "Hi Ca. Why aren't you up walking?" She looks disturbed; her attention somewhere else besides pacing. "Something's not right."

"Yes, I agree," the aide says.

"Let's see if we can find out what's wrong." I move the arm with red marks. "Seems okay."

I feel her feet; get no response. I feel along her legs look for bruises. I see some redness. I put one hand behind her knee, my other hand under her foot and lift.

"*Eeee!*" she yells.

Something is wrong.

"I'm going to speak to the nurse Cathy, please stay with her."

I tell the nurse what I saw, she gets Carol's records. "She was x-rayed after the fall," she says, "nothing's broken." Same words I heard on the phone. I explain how I lifted her foot and she yelled. This gets her attention; we go to Carol's room. Seeing Carol not able to lift her foot, the nurse agrees she's hurt. "It's probably the fall. I suspect bruises from the fall."

"I'd like another x-ray done."

"It can be done tomorrow morning; I'm sure they're gone by now."

"No. I want it done now," I persist, thinking, three o'clock shift change, worst time of the day.

"If you get me a wheelchair, I'll bring her down to radiology myself."

The nurse confirms my thoughts, shift change and no one in x-ray. "I'm not going anywhere until I find out what's wrong," I say. She finally calls downstairs and I hear, "Okay, she'll be right down."

125

The nurse, aide and I get her into a wheelchair while she makes noises but doesn't resist. Like an animal that knows it's hurt and needs help.

The radiologist meets us at the door.

"I x-rayed her already. Nothing showed." Again the words.

"Could you please x-ray both hips, knees, and ankles this time," I ask.

He helps me get her onto the cold, hard steel table. Her cries vibrate through me. I feel pain along with her. Eyes closed, she makes faces. I stroke her hair saying, "I promise after this is over, we'll get chocalotta ice cream, even if we have to rob the kitchen."

A few seconds later, the doctor comes out from his x-ray closet. "Her left hip is broken."

They x-rayed the wrong leg yesterday?

"Damn"—and grab hold of a chair to steady myself. "How could this happen?" I ask. "What do we do now? Where do we go from here?" Questions I remember from the support group, never related to me, always someone else asking. We'd all said, 'if a break, put them in a wheelchair and give pain medication.'

Now it's my decision. Not someone in the group.

I ask the doctor, "What would you do if it were your mother?"

"Because she's young and active, I'd fix it. They'll probably do a hip replacement."

After much indecisiveness, he makes the decision for me, and within an hour, Carol is on her way to the hospital. I stay behind collecting records, then get stuck in commuter traffic, playing relaxation tapes.

Twenty minutes after Carol's arrival in emergency, I give information to the clerk: health care surrogate, power of attorney all I keep with me. I see my friend tied to the bed yelling, "*Rata, Rata, Rata, Rata.*"

I feel sick, want to throw up, but instead ask the nurse, "Please untie her?"

"She can't get out of bed."

"She won't—I promise. But if you keep her tied down, she's going to keep yelling. I'll stay with her, she won't get out of bed." I help the nurse untie her wrists, and we are left alone.

I stroke her arm, and she looks at me. Her eyes full of sorrow. The nurse returns with a sedative.

Waiting seems an eternity. Finally by evening she's assigned a room and sleeps. I ask the floor nurse to make copies of all important papers. She assures me they will take good care of my friend. I feel better.

I watch her sleep out of pain. The nurse says nothing will be done tonight, it's too late. I make the sign of the cross on Carol's forehead, kiss her on the cheek, and leave. At the nurses' station I make sure they have my home phone number, in case there's a change in the middle of the night. Now, my drive is in darkness, over forty-five minutes, but the thought of myself stays away. I think *only* of Carol.

Home late, I call the nursing agency recapping what has happened, ask them to send an aide to the hospital instead of the nursing home. I eat a bowl of cereal and go to bed. I think of the day, praying she will be free of pain, sleeping.

The next morning, I call the hospital and speak with Carol's aide.

"How's she doing?"

"Sleeping since I got here at seven."

An aide Carol knows, I'm happy. If there's anything to be happy about? Carol has irregular heart beats. They're going to wait to operate, she tells me.

When at the hospital, I stop at the nurses' station to ask how Carol is. Not the same nurse as yesterday. She asks, "Are you family?"

"No, she's my friend."

"Well, we can only give information to family members."

I don't need this. The wrong hip x-ray is enough. Obviously, she hasn't seen the legal papers I left yesterday. I tell her I'm healthcare surrogate and to look at her records for necessary papers. I'm not wasting my time with closed minded people, and walk away.

Poor Ca, she's in a new place, can't pace, with new faces, and God knows what else. I call the doctor, he says nothing will be done until the heart stabilizes.

Five days later she goes for surgery. I go to early mass, then wait in her room. I call the agency saying I'll be there all day, not to send an aide until evening.

Four hours later, I hear that voice. "Rata, Rata, Rata, Rata." I smile thinking, Here she comes. Good for her, she made it.

She's brought in, awake. Two men transfer her to her bed as she speaks in that language.

I can't help but say, "She's speaking in tongues, you know. She got an in with *You Know Who*."

20

W hy can't she just walk? She *wants* to."

"She has to learn to stand before she can walk," says the therapist, "just like children learn to stand before they walk."

I feel for her. She's in a wheel chair now and stands in a wooden box up to her waist for therapy everyday. She stands a long time and soon her head rests on her folded arms. I think of grade school, when nap time came.

Weeks go by, phone calls come, "Carol fell out of the wheelchair, but she's all right. Just a few bruises." I listen, happy she's trying to walk; but when I see the bruises, I feel different—once more hurting for her.

Finally, I speak up, "Does she need to break something else before you do something? Can't you put something in front of the chair to stop her from falling out?"

"It's against regulations. We cannot restrain a patient," is the answer.

After many falls, a device called a *lap buddy* is attached to the chair—a piece of hard foam that also acts as a tray. She likes it, not only is it serving the purpose of keeping her from falling, she can also bang on it to get out her frustrations.

As long as Medicare pays for it, the 'standing box therapy' goes on. *For what reason? She isn't going to walk again, the simple reason, she's forgotten how.* Just what we'd talked of in the support group.

It's hard for me to understand. The woman I saw years ago, with that long stride, is not only captive in her mind but also captive in a wheelchair. That little bit of independence has been taken from her. *'How much more can she take? How much more does she have to go through for God to say, 'Enough!'* I want to yell, curse, rip everything apart, just as *she* did in the beginning years of the disease. It won't help, so I try to go on.

I take the written pages out of the drawer, and write of the hip break along with my anger. It's depressing and I return them to the drawer.

My lease of a year and a half is up. I have to leave the ocean. Fran, the realtor, tells me I can rent the other bedroom in her condo. *The same condo complex I lived with Carol. Do I want to go back there?* I have no choice. The money Mom left me is gone. I get $600 a month alimony and maintenance, maybe in years to come I can buy something. I'll pay Fran four hundred rent, buy food and maybe see a movie once in a while. Thank God I still have Carol's car.

I pack two suitcases, clean the bathroom, and take the *'Don't look forward'* message, putting it in my pocketbook. Other items have been brought to storage and I wonder if I'll ever see them again? My life's baggage is getting less. I sit on the balcony taking in the beauty. The ocean is calm, no whitecaps as the day I moved in. *"Goodbye,"* I whisper with a tear and a smile.

My next living space is small, a daybed, table, and chair—quite different from others I'd been used to. In fact, it reminds me of the bedroom I grew up in. It's light with morning sun, and Fran has put a new bed spread on. I can use the guest bathroom. I don't think of trivial things anymore, such as four bedroom, three bath colonials and country clubs.

I'm facilitator four years now at the support group, but above all, my driving is better. I'm not afraid. Fran is a lovely person, once in the ministry. I learn more of God. Our talks at dinner are how He influences our lives without us knowing, a tap on the shoulder every once in awhile to get our attention. How people are put in our path to smooth out the potholes and bumps along our journey. *We* make choices whether to walk around them or not. I'm learning, changing your thoughts can change your life.

In spring, a new woman visits the support group. She's opening an adult day care center in town and offers me a job. I say goodbye to my friends at the support group.

Before opening the center, days are spent working on monthly activity calendars. I think of things Carol and I did; play cards, puzzles, exercise, sing, dance, until she went downhill—maybe the job will be different.

We decide 'not' to call people patients. *Visitor* sounds friendlier. One visitor in a wheelchair, says she wants to take me home. I like her. Another visitor doesn't know what day it is and reminds me of Carol. 'What day is it? What day is it?' repetitive without combativeness. A gentleman visitor reads the paper or watches television. He's frail, his wife doesn't want him alone while she works. Loved ones from the support group come. I like this work. Seven-thirty to five, a mile and a half from home. I'm tired at the end of each day and have a feeling of accomplishment, serving others. *After all, isn't that why we're here? To look after our brothers and sisters so they won't feel alone?*

A year gone. I have to move. Fran's mother is ill, and she needs to sell the condo. *Where will I go?*

Sitting at the diner after work, in the classifieds I see a room for rent. It's in the old neighborhood not far from Sea Trail my first home. I call.

A young woman with long dark hair greets me at the door. "Rose?"

"Yes, hi," I feel I know her. "I'm happy to meet you Christina."

The room is large and clean. Something I could live in. "Would you like something to drink?" she asks.

"A glass of water will be fine, thank you." *Where do I know her from?*

For two hours, we sit in deep conversation about our ancestry. She's Greek. Her father brought his family to the United States when she was young. We chat like we've been reunited.

At eleven o'clock I tell her I need to work in the morning and have to go.

"I've enjoyed talking with you, Rose."

"Same here. I feel as if I know you."

"Me too," she says walking me to my car.

"Oh, I almost forgot. When can I move in?"

"I guess we forgot that detail. How about tomorrow?" taking a key off her key chain. "Come anytime you want. I'll be at work all day," handing me the key.

We say goodnight and I think on my way back to Frans, funny, how I feel I know her. A warmth comes over me, knowing I'll have a home again with someone 'I think' I know.

The next day after work I move in. First I tape the message in the medicine cabinet. Christina has put scented candles and flowers in the bathroom, welcoming me. *Nice*.

The days go fast, working, coming home, typing calendars, visiting Carol on the weekends. I sometimes see Debbi for counseling, but she's more of an old friend now. I'm living an almost 'normal' life.

Christina and I have fun deciding who's going to cook. We sit over cups of coffee discussing our backgrounds, how similar they are. I find we are alike in important areas, living life and the willingness to help others.

After a year, Christina's boyfriend comes from Greece, they decide to buy a house and raise a family. I say goodbye, giving them my love. "We'll stay in touch," we say.

My path leads me to a neighbor down the block—an older woman who's having difficulty making ends meet. It's amazing how my faith has grown, living the way I am.

My new roommate, Kathleen, is fourteen years older than me. Her daughter and grandchildren live next door, and it gives me a chance to see what my own children and their children might be doing now.

We don't have contact, because they choose not to. I send birthday and Christmas cards, but get no response. So

I honor their wishes, letting them live their own lives, kind of like my father and me after *he* moved to Florida. I never kept in touch with him, remembering how he treated me, and my mother. I guess the saying, what goes around comes around, is true, but I never treated *my* children with unkindness. I don't linger on this thought, it gets me down, and Lord knows I don't want to be down.

21

Another year gone. I'm working at an assisted living facility as activity director. The money isn't great, but I love it, plus I have health benefits.

My main idea is to keep residents out of their rooms. I want them up out of bed, moving their bodies and minds. Monday mornings, we're off to church, then back for chair exercises. Later I hand out juice and read the daily paper to them, not forgetting horoscopes. To one woman I read, "You're going to meet someone tall, dark, and handsome." And like fifth graders they laugh, teasing each other. I laugh with them.

We sit for table games: poker, dominoes, gin rummy, some play bridge and teach me. When lunch time comes, they'd rather stay in the activities room for more fun. I tell them, No it's time to eat and I'll see you at one-thirty for fun and games. Now go and enjoy your lunch.

"Aren't you going to eat?" some say, and "When will I know it's one-thirty?"

I reassure them I'm going to eat lunch and will knock on their doors when it's one-thirty.

I fill out the morning's activities report: who came, how they participated. 'Some, all, or none', keeping a daily log helps me know who doesn't attend activities. When done I join my coworkers for lunch and different conversation.

At one-thirty I knock on doors waking some from naps, "We're having a chat in the activity room. C'mon down," I say.

Some want to lie in bed, especially the new ones. They're afraid, feel out of place, but I keep after them. I want them with others, knowing they're not alone, and may have something in common with another.

Some I let stay in their rooms, because I know it's hard to join a group. Making time during the week, I visit them for quality time. They tell me they feel alone, left behind and I understand, not forgetting how I once felt.

Later in the afternoon we go for ice cream shakes, usually there's a lineup. They sign up at the front desk, but the van only holds six, so some have to stay home. Feelings are hurt when I say, "You went last week—we have to give someone else a chance."

"She's your favorite," I hear, and explain, to get back on their 'good side'.

On Tuesday mornings, we go shopping for personal items or just window shop. I remind George, the ninety-two year old, good looking Irish man, "Stay with the group, George." The women love when he dances and sings to them. He usually doesn't listen, but I remind him anyway.

After shopping he's no where to be found. With everyone in the van, I drive looking for him. Someone spots him walking out of the doughnut shop. I tell the group, when we pass George everyone wave goodbye. They snicker.

As we near George, everyone waves and smiles. He puts his palms toward heaven, as if saying, 'Hey, where are you going?' I back up, he gets in and I read him the riot act. "Don't you go and get lost like that. You scared me, and everyone else. Next time, you won't be allowed on the trip." He smiles. "George, I'm serious," I end with.

On the way back to the ALF, he asks to stop at the bank. Says he wants to cash a check.

"Do you have an account?"

"No."

"You need an account to cash a check. Why don't you let the facility cash it?"

"Take my word, they'll cash it. I'll bet you a nickel," he insists, in a singsong way.

"Okay, you've got a bet."

Arm and arm we walk into the bank. Nearing the tellers' window three women yell, "Hey George, where have you been? We've missed you!"

"You son of a gun, they know you," I say.

When he comes out, he grins saying, 'See, I told you I could cash a check'. I reach in my pocket, hand him a nickel, "It's only because you're so good-looking."

At the end of the day one activity is left, the men's outing. The guys want to go for ice cream. George, four guys and me order sundaes. They talk of when they were kids, and how expensive things were. I listen and learn.

The next morning, I find George has passed away during the night. I'm shocked because he was so healthy. He told me of speakeasies in New York he went to. How hard it was for him because his dad died young. He had to quit school, go to work to help feed his brothers and sisters. When his daughter came for his belongings, I met her in his room and told her how sorry I was.

"Rose, he loved to kid you. He woke towards the end, sat up, and said, 'N goes there'."

I laughed, telling her, "We played crossword yesterday, sounds like he had the right letter. I loved kidding him too. Your father made my days easier. Everyone loved him."

Knowing George, and the fun we had in activities, made me happy, learning things I didn't know. He enjoyed life to its fullest and spread it to others. 'George will be missed', someone said at his memorial the next day, held in the activity room.

I'd only been working a month, when Emma jumped into the pond, in front of the facility. After that, every time I went to Emma's room saying there's an activity going on, she'd shake her head vigorously, '*NO*'.

She usually read a book and spoke broken English due to a heavy German accent. I took it on myself to visit her a few minutes each day, whether she wanted me there or not. At times, she'd say, 'get out' and I'd leave, saying, "I'll see you tomorrow." After awhile she looked forward to my coming and confided in me. "What's the good of living if I can't see or hear? Look," pointing to a walker parked by the side of her chair, "I can't walk without that. I'm ninety-eight years old. What's left?"

"Well, you can't go anywhere. You know more than me, so you have to stay around and teach me."

She studies my face, shakes her finger and smiles. I knew I'd made a friend.

The other residents were not kind to her, because of her hardness, but we got along. I took her shopping, just the two of us. She liked that *special* attention. I saw her come out of her shell, and at 100 she was transferred to the nursing home confined to a wheelchair. On my way to and from lunch I'd stop to see her.

"Hi Emma, how you doing?" and listen for more wisdom.

She passed at 103.

At arts and crafts one day, I lay a white sheet of paper and magic markers on the table in front of my friends. I'd brought two music tapes from home, one classical—soft violins—the other, fast, pop music. They sit, questions on their faces.

"Today we're not going to paint birdhouses or make beaded flowers. We're going to see what we're about inside, our emotions. When you hear the music, I want you to take your marker and draw to the timing of the music."

Before I get the words out, I hear, "Oh, I don't want to do that," or "I can't do that," or "I don't know how to draw."

I tell them this is not about being better than anyone else or taking a test. It's about having fun. I want you to try, and I hit the play button, hoping there won't be anymore 'Ohs' and 'Ahs'.

Markers in hand, they go from dots and dashes to soft flowing lines, drawing to music. When done, we talk of the fun it was and next week we are going to have an art sale.

We sing, "Oh, we ain't got a barrel of money...," and my buddy, Carol, is with us in thought. I see *her* face in all these faces.

I've learned if I give myself to others it keeps me from thinking of my self. What's that saying? *It's much better to give than to receive.* I think God said it sometime, somewhere. My friends have taught me much about myself. I guess I'm no different from anyone else. I'm normal, after all.

22

In 2001 the first thing I do is tape, *Don't look forward He will look after you today, tomorrow, and always*...inside my new cabinet. Reading it, I must believe.

This is a different kind of move. I've taken my divorce savings and have rented a one/one condo, in a 55 and over community. It's all mine, no roommates. I have a door of my own. I buy a bed and lamp, that's it for now.

I've quit my job due to stress. My heart is acting up, doing those odd beats. Residents had told me things I wasn't happy to hear, like diapers weren't changed at night because the aide never came. Another worker confided, he got together with his friend and smoked Pot in back of the building.

I understand things are tough, but what's happened to, respect for your elders and the ill? Doesn't it mean anything anymore? I've come to believe Health Care is an *Industry* not a service. Oh, there are those who feel for others and serve well, but it needs fixing, not with a band-aid, but an overhauling from top to the bottom. Too many generals and not enough soldiers. Too many suits and ties, and nice dresses, while hands on people are underpaid and overworked. *When will it change?*

I go to thrift stores looking for used furniture and spot a couch.

"My God, it's *our* couch," I whisper to myself.

The same pink and green couch, with brown soil marks. It's hard not to cry, thinking when we sat and watched television on it, parties with friends and family. Good memories.

I wonder does it still have urine stains? And turn the cushion over. *Yep, still there. Poor Carol, she didn't know what was happening back then.*

I feel a piece of me sitting here, open for everyone to look at. I want to burn it, not have it exist, then decide to walk on through the store looking at other items. I say another goodbye.

I have a new feeling about me, a good one—a feeling of worth.

For years, I've given myself to dementia, Alzheimer's, stroke, and other forms. I'm tired and wish I were younger. I get calls from caregivers who live here, 'Can you come and stay with my wife while I go to the store?' and I go. I remember when *I* asked for help. Another call comes, 'My wife walked out of the house, I've called the police.' The neighbors form a search party, and find the woman in the next complex, safe.

It's like living in a large assisted living facility without the name or corporation behind it. Residents get together, play golf, go to the pool, exercise, play games, bingo, bridge; have parties at the clubhouse—so much to keep a person active. It's a community where everyone helps each other.

I see a golfer walk to the green pushing his walker. It has three wheels, just like the ones I saw working and in the nursing home. He's bent over, has a dowager's hump, possibly in his nineties. In the middle of his walker, a bag carries a few golf clubs. I watch him hit the ball, push his walker, hit the ball, push his walker. *What determination.* I want to yell, 'Put it in the hole—good for you, keep going forward!'

It's a happy place to live, even though I don't join in the activities. Everyone is in their seventies, eighties, nineties and more. I'm in my early sixties. I know though, I have a future here if I want it.

I find a new church, on my way to visit Carol one day, and meet Pastor Jim. I tell him of Carol and how she would have liked him. He listens of my visits with her and prays with me, that I may find my way and know that Carol is not in pain. I tell him, "Jim, I think Carol is no different from Jesus who suffered and cried out, 'My God, my God, why have you forsaken me? Take this cup from me.'" Jim lets me talk.

Unpacking items from storage that I haven't seen since 1995, I run across Carol's little black daily entry books—dates of her activities and appointments. I read them. I have the time now.

The pages are full of what she did each day and plans for the next…birthday cards to send and phone calls to make. She writes of the outside temperature, and how her back hurts after a golf game.

She leads me into the next day with every word. I touch the words—faded now, soft rolled-up page edges from age. I feel her here with me. My heart goes out to her as I read more about her before we met. I stumble across names we knew up north. Some words have no meaning; and then, I see words of me, times together at West Meadow Beach, golf courses, doctors' appointments, visits from friends and family, my gallbladder operation, EP study that diagnosed my heart palpitations.

I see something else behind her words. Her handwriting is different. The first years are clear, scrolled to the right, large soft strokes. Then came the illness, short, pointy, choppy strokes. Calm in the first books, then later, the anxious Carol. I recall times when she had trouble remembering, and see it in her writing. She tried hard to remember, with clues on pages to help her, *R* for Rose and *C* for Carol.

I come across her birth date February 14, circled *B,* for birthday. She's written the years 1992 minus 1926 to figure her age was 66. She writes of the beach club, names of people we met for her birthday lunch. She writes "lovely time + fun." Some clues are hard to read, as only Carol knew what they meant. There are golf dates on every page, TV times of golf tournaments, and hair appointments.

On January 27, she writes, 'Went to a movie.'

February 1991, '7:30 a.m. Dr. Mike, research center.'

August 22, 1992, she writes, 'Hurricane Andrew 110 mph off Florida, boarding up. Rose and I to friends' home.'

August 31, 1992, 'Auto train to Long Island.'

September 9, 1992, 'We see the house again and eat in Stony Brook.'

The books go on and on. I read her writing and remember the past, realizing I need to finish *my* writings, instead of putting them in a drawer.

23

I push the wheelchair forward, passing nurses, aides, and other residents. Behind me I hear, "There they go for ice cream. She comes every week. How sad." I smile, letting them know nothing's changed—the love is still there.

Valerie says, "How are you two today?" in broken English. *Eight years now.*

"We're fine, thank you—and you?"

"I'm fine—chocalotta, right?"

"Yes, one for my friend, please," and we laugh.

She hands me the ice cream, and we head outside for our quality time—our connecting time—our together-as-one time.

Bowl in hand, I push to the large shade tree so light won't bother her eyes. Inside every day, they don't know sunlight. Her right eye is shut for no medical reason, her face on that side drawn tight, making deep crevices in her cheek.

We'll face the pond today, watch the ducks. I put on the brakes. *As if she's going somewhere?* Place the bowl on a ledge, and drag a chair over for myself. Settled, I look for a smile...not yet...maybe later. She's been asleep since we left upstairs. Hoping to wake her, I start our song. "Oh, we ain't got a barrel of money, maybe we're ragged and funny, but we travel along, singing a song, side by side." No connection.

Singing, I remember the times we sang from Florida to New York. It made our trips shorter, and we didn't sound half bad.

Usually when I sing, she gives me a smile and winks. Not lately though, she sits and stares into space, and I pray I'm not losing total contact with her, for that little bit makes me feel again. *Oh, how that little look would lighten my heart today.* Sometimes I think I hear, 'I'm a prisoner in this body and I long to play the game of golf again.'

"Kaditchka, open your eyes," I say. "You have such beautiful eyes, let me see them." I stroke the side of her face. It takes a while, but soon she opens them, she's alert.

I remember the first time I gave her the name, *Kaditchka,* many years ago when she told me her grandmother came from Germany. Why I picked the name, I'll never know—just a fun thing to do back then. While working in the condo, I'd say, "Kaditchka, what do you want to eat?" and she'd laugh. Now I use it hoping to bring back a memory.

I put a little ice cream on the tip of the spoon, touch her lips with it. She wrinkles her nose, squishes her lips, as if it's lemon. Finally I get some into her mouth, she realizes what it is and wants more. She eats fast. I want it to last for *my* sake. I love seeing her eyes open, aware of something simple, like ice cream. I know once it's gone she'll be off *somewhere* else.

She finishes. I stroke her hair and tell her of friends who say hello and golf tournaments on television. She closes her eyes.

I let her sleep so I can cut her fingernails. They've gotten long. The aides have trouble cutting them, because she clasps her hands tightly together. I guess her strength comes from gripping a golf club for so many years. I undo her wrapped around fingers that have now latched onto my hand—another contact we have. She makes faces and movements with her head—sudden jerks. I talk and sing as I clip, feeling there's just two of us. No one else exists. *We are in our space.*

When done, I sit back and look at her. Her hands are wrinkled, have spots, red-blue and purple. They're no longer tan from sun.

She's shorter, bent to one side and cannot pull herself up to a sitting position. Her face also has that red-purple tint. Her lips are dry, white and wrinkled, no life, no blood circulating. She dribbles and has no teeth from years of grinding them. Her feet and ankles are swollen. Her legs are bent and stiff, and when I try to straighten them to put a shoe on, I'm sure she's in pain, by the expression on her face. She has scales on her skin, no longer the beautiful bronze tan. She no longer smells of baby oil she used for tanning, but reeks of urine and other odors. I tell the aides she needs changing, and they say, "Yes, okay," and go on with something or someone else, like when I worked. I only hope it gets done later.

Her hair is in disarray, the beautician has bleached it blond even though I've asked not to. No one listens—because they want to do it 'their' way. I let it go, don't get angry anymore. She has scales on her scalp, aides put gel on, I've asked not to. I've written letters, spoken to supervisors, but no one listens. I've given up.

The curves on her body are points, from great weight loss. Her ribs show under the blouse she wears and her neck stiff, with great hard cords from trying to hold up her head. It dangles to one side, like a ball on a string.

Her shoulders are bent forward and her hips large because of double diapers. To change her, they use a machine called a hoist to get from chair to bed. I don't watch, I can't bare the pain on her face.

It's two-thirty—time to bring her upstairs for a nap—but first, four hands are joined as one, and the Lord's Prayer is said, *by one*.

24

In 2002, instead of my usual visit before lunch, it's three-fifteen and Carol's on the toilet being held by the machine I hate.

Belts cut deep under her arms. I ask Nora, a new aide, to take her off the toilet.

"Not now, I'm too busy."

"Her arms are turning blue from the belts."

Again, No, that it's good for her to sit on the toilet.

Carol is agitated. So, like old times I kneel on the floor.

Twenty minutes later I'm at the nurses desk. Someone new. *They change workers like toilet paper.* Her tag reads, 'Jean'.

"Excuse me Jean, my friend Carol, in room 219 has been on the toilet a long time. Her arms and hands are turning purple," pleading.

She also says it's good to sit on the toilet. I retreat to Carol's room, make myself busy straightening her closet. Clothes are all over the floor, I hang them up. A large bag type purse sits on the dresser.

"What the heck is this doing here?" talking to myself. I do that a lot these days.

I know it's not Carol's and am sure it isn't her roommate's. She's like Carol, can't speak or walk.

The bag's open, showing a plastic bag full of orange prescription bottles. I go to the administrator's assistant, Maureen. I've known her since '94. She's helped me with past problems. Her secretary tells me to go right in.

"Hi Maureen."

"Hi Rose, how are you?"

"Not so good right now. There's a bag full of prescription bottles on Carol's dresser. With Alzheimer's patients walking around getting into things, I don't think it's a good idea for it to be there."

She looks at me, writes something down and thanks me. She'll handle it, she says. I leave.

Back upstairs Carol's still on the toilet. I look at my watch, ten to four, over half an hour. God knows how long before I came. Her right arm is purple.

In the hall I spot Nora coming out of another room. "Nora, I want Carol off the toilet, now!"

"You can't speak to me like that. I have others to take care of."

"Carol's arm is purple!" I persist.

She continues saying it's okay and it will come back to its normal color.

"Nora, I know you have a hard job. I worked in health care, also. I know it's hard work, but this is ridiculous. Will you please take my friend off the toilet?"

She looks at me, then asks me to wait in the hall while she goes into Carol's room.

I sigh, finally, not believing some of the things that go on. It doesn't make sense—but then it never did. I'm sure it has something to do with the shift change. Time for one to leave, another to take over. What would happen if they worked beyond their clock out time? When I worked the aides would line up near the clock, because they weren't allowed to work over time, except if they were asked to.

While waiting, a woman comes out of the director of nurses' office, goes into Carol's room, closes the door. Minutes later she comes out holding the large, bag/purse. She passes me, and I can't resist saying, "I don't think it's safe to have that around, do you?"

She shakes her head, 'no,' annoyed. But I know Maureen got my message across.

A male aide goes into the room. Help Nora remove Carol from the hoist, I think.

Ten minutes pass. I wonder, what they're doing? I go in, see Nora slowly running a brush through Carol's hair, two aides conversing in another language—*not Carol's.*

"I'll do that, Nora. Thank you very much. I'd like to take my friend outside, now." The male aide leaves, followed by Nora.

I take Carol downstairs. I'm so afraid the aides will take their revenge out on her when something like this happens. It's happened so many times in the past, and wonder if the bruises came from aides who were too heavy handed with her?

Being late, no one is manning the ice cream parlor. I get a cup from the main kitchen. We sit under the shade tree till she falls asleep. I notice blood running from her nostril, and take her upstairs. Report it to the nurse.

Nothing's changed in all the years. The aides have too much to do and not enough time to do it in.

The nursing home nightmares go on....

One Sunday, I can't remember which year, because my weekly visits blend into *one* horrible nightmare, I enter the dining room and see an aide feeding Carol. I tell the aid, I'll feed her, if she wants to help others.

Carol's agitated at something. Usually, because something's bothering her—she's wet, hungry, or just unable to communicate.

I feed her the ground-up yellow/green stuff—a casserole they say—along with applesauce, which she loves. I alternate 'yellow/green' stuff, applesauce. She has thickened fluids, apple juice and water. I'm sure she doesn't get enough liquid, her lips are dry and cracked. The same when I worked, *they* become dehydrated.

The dining room's noisy, filled with agitation among the patients. Something's bothering them. One patient is walking out the door.

An aide yells from across the room, "Sit down in your chair, Evelyn. You know you can't go out alone."

"I'm not alone, I'm with her," Evelyn points to another woman coming in the doorway and repeats, "You're never alone—you're never alone— you're never alone." Over and over, as Carol used to. I feel it's being said for me.

When finished eating, I bring her to her room, comb her hair, then down for chocolate ice cream. She's happy, her face has a smile. In my mind I hear, *Thank you.*

I bring her outside to get air in her lungs and have our quality time. A *flutterby* joins us. She doesn't see it, her head is slumped down; but I know it's here for both of us, a beautiful spirit has come to say hello. Soon, she's asleep, as her head drops further, her body twitches, just as it has since the beginning of the disease.

Back upstairs, I tell her I love her and make the sign of the cross on her forehead as I've done for so many years.

Passing the nurses' station, I tell the nurse, "She smells, I think she needs changing. Thank you. I'm heading home now. Have a good day."

In the elevator I hit number one and look down at the floor. The doors close. I haven't looked back in a long time. I don't want my last look of her to be sitting alone in a wheelchair.

It's the day before Thanksgiving, I'm feeling nothing— no sadness, no happiness, no feelings. Like living in a vacuum. I try to put the idea of another holiday out of my mind. I'm better when I don't think of holidays. I've noticed for years I cope better when there's no one around. There's too much emphasis placed on holidays. Every day should be a holiday as it was when Carol and I lived together to life's fullest. I dread them because of the fibs I have to tell. "Oh, a friend invited me for Thanksgiving dinner," or "I'm going to my brother's."

Usually, I visit Carol, then go to a movie to be among people I don't know, and watch *them* have fun.

Another Christmas has come, Carol's slumped over to one side as usual, her eyes closed.

An aide brings Carol's food tray and says hello. I undo the saran wrap that covers the hot, pureed meal with thickened drinks, as usual.

She sleeps while I arrange food. Broth over pureed food, so it's easier for her to eat. I ask, "How about some peaches to start with?" rubbing her cheek lightly to wake her. I've never stopped talking to her. I want her to know I'm here.

She doesn't open her eyes, but I know she's awake—just something you learn after being around someone for so long. The peaches touch her lips, she opens her mouth. Memories of feeding my children come when they were very young. I study her face, see pain. Sometimes, it's like this, then she's better after a while. *Maybe it's the pain of hunger?*

I start our song, *Barrel of Money*, and get no response. When this happens, I wonder why she needs to go through this hell.

What's the purpose of it—for me to see how one I love has deteriorated, and someday soon will never be? Years of this makes no sense.

Through the forty-five minute meal, she opened her eyes once to look at the aide across from us, feeding another patient.

"Ca, it's time for chocalotta ice cream." She smiles—or am I seeing something that isn't there?

I tell the nurse, "I'm going to cut her nails in her room, then we're going for ice cream."

"Okay, have fun—see you later," the nurse replies.

After clipping her nails, I get a jacket from the closet and drape it around her, it's chilly today.

The ice cream parlor isn't open yet, we head outside where other residents are sitting in the sun. There is a private birthday party, in the corner of the building where residents are having fun singing.

Her eyes are closed. She looks asleep. I see her white hands. *This is what a dead person's hands look like.* I hate the thought, but it's there.

We sit in the sun. I whisper, "This will be good for your chest congestion." She sleeps while I listen to sounds around us, birds, then a flutterby comes to say hello. I remember that first one on Long Island playing golf. 'Hello Flutterby,' she'd said, like it was yesterday.

I bring her upstairs and find a cup of chocalotta ice cream in the dayroom. I set her in front of the birdcage, in case she opens her eyes, then she will see the birds on the floor of the cage. I put a teaspoon to her lips. She opens her mouth to take her favorite food. I ask the nurse how Carol's doing.

She shakes her head—"She's failing"—words I've heard since the hip break. "Everyone has colds and coughs."

"Please take good care her," I tell the nurse, and kiss Carol. She never opened her eyes.

She has her eyes closed all the time now, except sometimes at ice cream time, when she opens them for a moment.

Valerie's at her post. "I'm sorry, we have no chocolate today," she says before I ask. "We have vanilla cheesecake."

"What do you think of vanilla cheesecake, Ca?" as if she's going to answer. *Funny, she's probably annoyed there's no chocalotta.*

She looked at me once today as I got up to throw away the napkin, I used to wipe her mouth with. When I came back, it startled her, and both eyes opened. She looked straight at me surprised, smiled, then closed them.

Someone once told me, *they* keep their eyes closed because they're getting ready to cross over to the other side, then they will have no recognition of what's here—*me*.

She's ill all the time, urinary infections, colds, or viruses. Today, I wheel her to the main cafeteria where I get something to eat. I fill my plate with a few pieces of lettuce, some beets, and some pink dressing. I place her near the window opposite me.

People pass, smile, probably thinking we're sisters. In a sense, we are. I eat fast, to get away from the area. Couples enjoy one another here. It's not like Carol's floor where everyone's in another world, speaking another language. People here are just elderly, can't take care of themselves, but have most of their wits about them. They'll soon play bingo, or listen to someone play the piano in the music room, like Carol used to do.

It's hot and humid outside, and it's only May. I feel old, tired and spent today, or maybe I do everyday. My life is here with her. I *have* no other life.

The drive home is long, without feeling—a death has come over me.

I stop at an ice cream shop near home for *my* chocolate ice cream soda. I drink it, going over the day's events. I can't dislodge myself from the nursing home. It takes hours, sometimes days, to get it out of my system.

I am late this Sunday getting to her. I stayed at church for coffee and cake with the parishioners.

Signing in, I round the corner near the ice cream parlor, see long buffet tables, draped in white cloths with different foods. Partway down the hall, I notice new faces—workers. I take the elevator. I head for the dining room, she isn't there, then look in the dayroom—not there either. *Please don't let her be sick in bed.* No call came that she was ill.

Her door is open. She's in bed looking one with the mattress. *What's the matter with her?* I try waking her, but she's in that other place, better than this one. I feel her forehead, not warm. I check her pulse, steady. *Why is she in bed?*

Walking back to the dining room I ask one of the aides if Carol's eaten lunch. She doesn't know.

Every worker looks new, *What's happening?* Then remember, it's a holiday—not my own—that's why different foods and decorations downstairs. Carol's floor has nothing, all regular aides are missing.

A woman dressed in a black suit asks, "Can I help you?"

"Yes, I'm Mrs. Lamatt, Carol Beinbrink's friend. She's in bed. Is she ill?"

The woman looks surprised, caught off guard, for lack of a better word. "Oh…Yes. I'll find out"—and excuses herself.

I wait in Carol's room. The woman never returns. Terra, a regular, I've known for years comes in.

"What's wrong with Carol? Why isn't she up?"

"Everyone's working downstairs. We didn't have a chance to get her showered and dressed this morning."

Did she eat breakfast? but don't ask. I've been let down too many times. I'm done making scenes. Yelling for years got me nowhere. It never changed a thing, and upset me. I knew this was the *health care industry*, just another nursing home nightmare.

"Would you please fix a lunch tray for her and I'll feed her in her room."

Terra apologizes. I tell her, I understand. Another aide comes to help get rid of Carol's stench while I wait in the hall. Minutes later she's propped up in bed, awake, smelling better. Terra brings lunch and leaves. The tray holds pureed foods. She's eager to eat. Or, is it that she didn't receive breakfast? I sing while feeding, the usual.

A new nurse comes giving her pain medication—two kinds now—she's quickly asleep. *When I'm not here, does she get fed?*

No chocolate anything today—the first in years.

Leaving her room, I see her roommate in the hall waiting for someone to help her. Like Carol, she's unable to hold up her head and keeps her eyes shut, but you know she's awake, you hear her grinding her teeth.

Tears come on my way to the ice cream shop. I remember the love we had, how we drank sodas long ago. I go to the movies, like every Sunday.

Months have passed, I see Carol today and bring her into the dayroom to feed her. The wheelchair is still in the upright position instead of tilted back. "We'll tilt the back," said the doctor, "keep pressure off her spine," but it's not—*what else is new?*

The Sound of Music is on television. I hear the song *Edelweiss* and think of past times when *we* sang it. I sing it now to wake her. I remember John playing it on the piano. We sang it when I worked.

Her head leans against the pad of the chair, slanted down. I try waking her, lifting her head, rubbing her cheeks and arms. It takes time to arouse her, which means they're giving her heavier doses of pain medications. She's also on antibiotics for a bladder infection, since the urine sample showed a 'strange organism.' Information will come tomorrow when I see the doctor.

She wakes when I put dessert to her lips. She still comes alive when sweets are offered. I feed her pureed turkey, stuffing, and potato, alternating sweet, so she'll keep eating. She drifts in and out of sleep. After an hour she's eaten a quarter of her food. I make sure she drinks the water and cranberry juice.

She stares at me, a look of anger. I sit back in my chair, look deep into her eyes and hear her *not* say, 'Rose, why do you want to keep me alive? For me, or for you?'

What am I doing? I feed her saying, good girl, after a spoonful, for what reason? She's not going to get better unless God steps in and changes things. So why do I want her to finish a meal?

I stop feeding her realizing it *is* for me. I watch her head rest against the pad. You can't even find a comfortable place to rest your head. Maybe tomorrow when I see the doctor, I'll mention it to him. Maybe I'll ask if you can be put on a larger dose of medication. Then you can sleep, have that look of pain gone from your face.

Maybe tomorrow I will ask....

25

2003

It's eleven at night. I've gotten up for a glass of milk, and fall into a wall, dizzy. I climb back in bed waiting for it to pass. It doesn't. Fear creeps in, no roommate in another bedroom. I'm alone, feel it in body and spirit. I reach for the blood pressure cuff in my nightstand. Years ago the doctor said, 'Keep track of your pressure and heart rate.'

It's up—higher than ever, 180/160. The machine must be wrong. I take it again. It doesn't change, more fear piggy backs onto the first. I take a tranquilizer. My head feels as if it's going to explode, shades of the sixteen year old.

It may not be a panic attack. It's been so long I've forgotten what they're like, but it's not my usual attack. My heart's beating fast but not out of rhythm.

I dial Mary, a friend I met at church. She's on the other side of town. She answers and I know I've woken her.

"Rose? What's the matter?"

"I think something's wrong."

"Yeah—what?"

"Well…uh…my blood pressure's up and I'm very dizzy. I'm afraid to call 911, if it's just a panic attack."

"You don't sound right to me. I'm calling 911."

"No, please don't. Can't you come over? I'm sure I'll be all right if someone's here."

"No! You need help...hang up. I'm calling now."

I take a deep breath, "Okay."

Maybe this *is* a good idea—but what about health insurance? *I don't have any.*

I foresee the paramedics breaking in the kitchen window. It's late, and I don't want to disturb the neighbors. Getting to a sitting position, I hold my head. It spins, as on a carnival ride. I close my eyes, better, get up, feel along the bedroom wall into the hallway to unlock the door. Eyes still closed I walk like a drunk back to bed.

Waiting, I do relaxation exercises, it doesn't help. The room spins.

The phone rings, a young woman asks, "Mrs. Lamatt?"

"Yes."

"This is the fire department. Your friend called saying you're not well. What's the matter?"

"I'm dizzy, can't stand without falling into walls. I'm not good at all."

"Stay in bed, the medics are on their way. Is your address 140 North Elder Road?"

"Yes. I've unlocked the door for them."

"Good, do you want me to stay on the line until they arrive?"

"No, I think I hear them now, thank you."

Someone's yelling, "HELLO, MS. LAMATT?"

"Yes, I'm in the back bedroom."

A young woman with long blond hair and a young man with large muscles come in my bedroom. They introduce themselves, quickly I forget their names. They're dressed in dark blue shirts, short sleeved and dark blue pants with red and white emblems on their sleeves and chest pockets.

"How're you doing?" one asks.

"Not too good."

I lift my head to greet them, but quickly slide back down. "Oh—very dizzy. The room is spinning."

"Stay still, I'm going to check your blood pressure and pulse," says the woman while the young man clamps a clothespin-type gadget on my finger.

"I'm checking your oxygen level," he says.

Both ask questions of past history. The medic reads off numbers 174/140. "Do you have a history of high blood pressure?"

"No. I take an anti-arrhythmic drug, for ventricular tachycardia."

"I notice a rhythm disturbance. I think you should go to the hospital," says the woman.

"But I…don't have health insurance."

At that, the man turns, to walk out.

"Are you really leaving?"

Looking back at me, laughing, he says, "Ms. Lamatt, my mother doesn't have health insurance. The hospital will take you, don't worry."

Mary comes in, I thank her for calling 911 and ask if she will go to the hospital with me. I'll meet you there she says.

Transferred to a canvas chair I'm taken down the outside steps. Eyes shut, it keeps the dizziness down. I ask Mary to lock the door and turn out the light.

In the ambulance, the woman checks my vitals. "Your blood pressure's still high. You'll feel a little stick. I'm putting an IV in," she says. "Think of your breathing, try to control it."

I try but can't focus.

They've called ahead alerting the hospital of a sixty-one year old female with dizziness, high B/P, throwing PVCs. I remember the same words years ago.

When there, the emergency room doctor asks questions, while the nurse hooks me up to a heart monitor and oxygen. I tell the doctor the same as the paramedics. "VT, no high blood pressure, but do throw PVCs once in a while."

The doctor asks questions of family.

"My brother lives here but he's on vacation in Europe." I think of the other so-called family member living at the nursing home. She couldn't help.

Blood work taken, in minutes the results are in the doctor's hands.

"Your blood work shows signs of small clots, somewhere in the body."

Hearing this, I think of Mom dying of a massive stroke. Working in health care, I knew clots traveled to heart, lungs, and brain. I'm afraid, yet feel confident I'm in good hands.

"Do you think it's a stroke?" I ask.

"I won't know till other tests are done," and he calls for brain and lung scans to be done. At three, reports are back. No clots anywhere.

They want to keep me overnight. Embarrassed, I say, "I don't have health insurance." They pay no attention.

At 6 a.m., I'm taken to a room upstairs. My blood pressure's dropping. I'm feeling better. I'm comfortable in *this* hospital. The one I've been in so many times, with Carol and without.

The next day, the doctor recommends seeing an ear, nose, and throat doctor, plus neurologist. Again, I say 'no health insurance,' again it doesn't matter. I'm the only one thinking of the cost. Where is the money going to come from? Also, in the back of my mind are the words I'd heard downstairs in emergency: *small clots*. Where were they?

For three days I'm tested, CTscans, MRIs, ultrasounds—and I keep repeating, "I don't have health insurance," no one's interested.

Pastor Jim visits, saying, "God will provide" and we pray together. I laugh with him, not worried.

On the third day I'm allowed to go home, still dizzy, no diagnosis, except small clots, none found. I'm given a new medication for dizziness. Meniere's Disease they say.

Once home, in the bathroom I study the saying attached to my medicine cabinet, *Don't look forward...Believe the words, Rose.* It's good to be home in my own bed. Other than tired, slightly dizzy, I feel pretty good. I'll watch a half hour news, turn the light out, and say a prayer of thanks to have a place to come home to. Tomorrow I'll finish the chapter I've been working on.

26

W hat the heck is that?" I wake, sitting on the porch in the rickety old web chair. In a tree at eye level, I see a tiny gray bird. Two of them, causing leaves to fall, bringing me back to the present with a grin.

I've never seen this type before, and run for the bird book. Scanning pages, I come across similar birds but not exact. *Boy, I wish Ca were here, she'd find it.* She's not, so I shelve the book. I'll have cereal tonight, and maybe ice cream to celebrate the new sighting with no name.

Church tomorrow—then a visit to Carol. I haven't been in a while. Hopefully I won't be dizzy. Typing all day, I'm tired and need rest. Time is sliding by too fast. I have to finish the book.

The day starts dizzy, weaving my way to the bathroom. In the shower, the curtain moves as I bend down to pick up the bar of soap that's fallen. I feel my heart pound in my head and ears. I better make it out of here before the paramedics find me this time naked. That wouldn't be a pretty sight.

In the kitchen I down an equilibrium pill, a diuretic, and heart medication with juice. Within the hour I'm better. I should know not to take a shower on an empty stomach, and no meds. You'd think I'd be smarter.

Driving to church, I think of when I was a child, kneeling between my parents, watching the priest give communion. I always admired priests because they were allowed to give communion. Women couldn't do this when I was young. Thank God, for changes.

Once there the preacher speaks of gifts we have to give to others, "Those of you who have singing voices, sing and praise God; those of you who are good with words, preach His word."

What gift do I have?

In the middle of the service, communion time comes, a chalice filled with grape juice and a plate with pieces of bread. The minister has consecrated it into the Body and Blood of Christ. That's when I realize the gift I hold. The same gift the priest offered me over fifty years ago when I made my first Holy Communion. I now have it to give. People from the congregation come to eat and drink. I offer the best gift of all—the Bread of Life.

My thoughts driving to Carol are not feelings of dread, seeing a body slumped over in a wheelchair. My thoughts are different. I thank God for the pain she's gone through, so I can feel the pain with her. The fear on her face I understand. I give thanks for the awareness that she is not alone; therefore, I am not alone, here, now, or ever. This is what love is—to feel what another feels. Love never dies, so we never die. This is the purpose of life. I finally know why I'm here: *There but for the grace of God, go I.* It's a comfort to have—a joining of minds. We have only to serve. We're here to be happy, enjoy life with our fellow human beings, not lonely and sad.

Carol is in the dining room waiting to eat, her head down, upper body to one side. It doesn't bother me. It's just the way it is. The aide is feeding her roommate.

"Hi Mike, how are you?"

"Hi, I haven't seen you in a while."

"I haven't been here. I've been sick with vertigo."

"Oh, that's no fun. I'm sorry."

"How's my girl today?" then turn to her, "Hello Kaditchka, how are you?" kissing her on the head.

She turns toward me, eyes wide open, smiles, almost a laugh.

"Hey, look at that. She recognizes you," Mike says.

I'm stunned. I haven't seen this since I can't remember when. So alert, as if she *does* know me.

"Mike, I think I'll feed her in the dayroom, if that's okay?"

"No problem, let me get you a tray. I'll bring it to you."

"Thanks, Mike, I appreciate it."

I maneuver her large wheelchair around others to the dayroom. I place her by the large window, so sun will shine on her body.

"You need that bronze tan you used to have, Ca." Again she looks at me as if she knows what I'm saying.

She's on a program for the terminally ill, with lots of people looking after her. The nurse called during the week telling me her vitals, saying she's down to 118. I'm forty pounds more than her.

I feed her thickened cranberry juice first, she opens her mouth. "Good girl," I say, and hate it, but it comes automatically. Pureed turkey, potatoes, green beans, and vanilla cake are next.

I sing our song, "Oh, we ain't got a barrel of money." She stares at me smiling, while chewing. She hasn't chewed in a long time. She'd been storing food in her mouth like a chipmunk, not swallowing, common when the swallow muscles don't work well. On a roll, I shovel it in, singing, then run out of songs.

"Ca, what would you like to hear?" She stares at me trying to talk. I can't believe this.

"C'mon, Ca, tell me what you want to hear. Tell me. I know, how about something we used to sing in church." I start, "Let there be peace on earth and let it begin with me." She smiles, making sounds as if she's singing *with* me. Happiness runs all through me.

Later, on our way for chocalotta ice cream, we pass the nurses' station. I put my hand to my mouth and whisper, "We're going downstairs to run around the block and get some ice cream. And if Carol lets me, I'll cut her nails."

The nurse puts her arm around my shoulder, "You're good to come and see her."

It's not a case of being 'good'. I want to see her. She's my friend. Don't they know that by now?

Off the elevator I'm happy, jumping for joy, she's smiled at me, tried to talk and sing with me. What more could anyone ask for? I'm ecstatic. I want everyone I pass to know. I smile at other caregivers when they pass us in the halls.

We see our old friend Valerie, with the treats—*ten years now.*

"No chocalotta today, bing cherry or pistachio."

"Oh boy, I'll have to take the nuts or cherries out; otherwise she'll choke," I say.

"I'll scoop around the side of the container so you won't have many. That should help."

"Thanks, Valerie, that'd be great. Give us cherry."

Carol's eyes are wide, watching, listening, taking it all in.

Seated, I feed her. "Boy, she sure is alert today. I haven't seen you in weeks. Where have you been?" asks Valerie.

I tell her of my illness, and Carol eats. When finished, I say, "Goodbye, we'll see you next week, God willing."

It's drizzling, too windy for our outside quiet time. I need to cut her fingernails. They're long, haven't been cut since I was here. We settle for the enclosed balcony. Seated I face her, taking scissors from my purse, ones she gave me long ago.

I unclasp her hands, she relaxes them for me to clip. I'm in awe how the visit's going. "Thanks Ca, for being awake. I love you." and clip. When done, four hands are joined, and The Lord's Prayer said, "Our Father who art in heaven..."

Almost asleep, I make the sign of the cross on her forehead. I take her inside, and park her next to the birdcage where it's quiet, all she can hear are birds chirping in conversation. If she wakes she'll see them, knowing she's not alone.

I tell the nurse all we've done and to have a good week.

"You also," she says.

In the elevator, I turn to see her head down. *God bless you, Ca.* The doors close.

Walking to the car, my step has a spring in it. I feel everything's right with the world. "Thanks Ca, for a beautiful visit. Thank you, God, for the gift of Carol. This is what it's all about, isn't it? We don't need anything but to show the gift of Your Love. That's what You gave me today. You showed me Your Love through Carol. Thank you." I talk to myself, but somehow I know I'm being listened to.

Driving home, serenity and all-is-right-with-the-world stays with me. I had given the gift of new life in church, and Carol had given me the gift of love. I sleep easy.

In the morning, ringing wakes me. I reach for the phone next to my bed and say, "Hello?"

"Hi, Rose. I think you should come." Jan from the nursing home.

Dressing, I think of yesterday, how she laughed, tried to talk to me. She recognized me. Driving, I think, this was something I thought about all the time. I'd prepared for it for years. I knew the call would come one day. I'd wanted it for so long. *Just like her to go and do it this way after yesterday.*

I've been sitting along side her bed for awhile, holding her hand. The nurse has given her Morphine. She stirs but not the way she used to, no sudden jerks. No clinging onto my hands. Her hands are cold. Her face calm, almost a smile. Blue has come to her fingernails and around her lips. She's leaving me this time in a different way. I play with the 'rose' on the chain around my neck, as I've done for years. The comfort it's given me. I think back to when I gave it to her, our first Christmas, then when she tried to destroy it. The 'rose' has seen a lot.

With eyes closed, I pray she's out of pain, free from this awful disease. Then think of good times; playing golf, walking the beach searching for shells, Geech, flutterbys, that contagious laugh she had. She made me laugh, even when I didn't want to.

A hand on my shoulder breaks my thoughts, "Rose? She's gone." I turn to Jan. I don't say anything, she knows how I feel and leaves us.

I stare at the beautiful face I knew so well. Tears make their way out the sides of my eyes, run down my cheeks. My sleeve catches them before they fall. I stay and stay, then think, there's nothing left. It's done. I get up, kiss her forehead, make the sign of the cross in that same spot.

Days later I'm happy, knowing she's free, then crying, knowing I'll never see her face again.

The funeral home calls, her ashes are ready for pick up. Going for them, fear and sorrow come, even though I know where I'll scatter them. I'll do it tomorrow at sunrise, but something gnaws at me not to wait.

Early evening, I walk along the wooden walkway to the sandy beach in front of Sea Trail. The sky gun-metal gray, meets the ocean. Approaching the water, I notice a pale pink spot on the edge of the horizon. I hold the heavy cardboard container under my arm, along with a beach chair from the car trunk and walk forward. Once at water's edge, I sit removing my socks and sneakers.

The outgoing tide is rough. I think how beautiful it still is after all these years, when she first brought me here.

I stare at the ocean, praying, ask God to take her, hold her forever. I pray for strength, then open the container. Inside is a plastic bag full of ashes. Carefully I take the bag out, loosen the twist tie around it. I head into the water. It's warm. I wade up to my calves, like years ago.

Opening the bag, I see her ashes, beige in color, not what I expected. I thought they'd look like ashes in a fireplace; these are like sand with pieces of bone. *Why did they leave bone for me to see?*

Bending over, I spread her to the left of me, thinking, This isn't her. Why are you sad? She's with God already.

As soon as they hit the water, they sparkle. Then like darting fish, are gone.

Looking out, I think of the day she swam far out and I called her back. Not this time.

"Go, Ca, you're finally free."

Tears run again, reality. I walk to the beach chair, sit, watch the ocean and sky, thinking she *is* free, part of nature now. To the right, a rainbow starts. I watch as it joins the pink spot at the horizon.

A gift—letting me know she's joined with God. Then another rainbow forms above the first—two rainbows now. Happiness inside me wants to burst out. I want to laugh and cry at the same time. I want to shout, tell everyone. After awhile I settle down letting the beauty remain in me, soaking me up. No person could make this happen. I know it's from God.

Soon it starts to drizzle. I pick up the chair, my sneakers and socks, and head for the car. Walking back along the wooden walkway, I look over my shoulder to see if the rainbows are still there. On my last look, they have faded and I know Carol has fulfilled her Journey.

I throw the now empty container in the garbage can and climb in the car. I sit a while; *Now what? Go home and make dinner? Carry on as usual?*

Days later it hits, what *do* I do now? All I've known for fourteen years was to worry and care for you. Now there's no one in a nursing home to look after, no other body to look after, except my own. How do I take care of *myself*? Taught as a child by my mother, in church, and school— it's better to give than receive. I've lost myself giving to others. How do I get my *self* back?

Just a Word

Epilogue

I had a hard time with Carol's illness, and realized only much later, how lucky I was to go through that part of her life with her. Believe me, I wanted that plate passed from me many times, but God let it go in His way, and in His time.

For readers who question whether Carol and I were gay? When I first saw Carol coming up the eighteenth fairway some eighty yards away, I truly was unable to move, I could not think, and she *did* hold my gaze. Time, in slow motion or possibly time stopped, is a better definition. All I saw was beauty, a sight I'd never seen the likes of before, and probably will never see again. I didn't know her when I saw her, but felt I had always known her. It's hard to explain and don't know if anyone *could* explain it. As I said in the story, she was someone I knew from way back, or always knew. It's a feeling you wouldn't know, unless you had experienced it yourself. I had read about her in my teens and early twenties. The newspapers wrote she was one of the best golfers on Long Island. I wasn't that big on golf and my boyfriend/husband took me to play once a year after we married. He knew of her, and had caddied at the clubs she played. Not until Joeie had said her name, did I realize she was the person in the newspapers.

I got away from the question, Were we gay? When you think of it, *gay* is also 'just a word'. I want to say 'no' to the question because I hate being classified in a group, but I will say 'no' with a possible 'yes'. I loved her beyond anyone I'd loved before, or maybe I had *never* loved before. And I'm pretty sure she loved me. I know she liked me, and I liked her. That's probably the important part—we liked each other—me, enough to give up my life for her, if I had to. And sometimes caring for her, I thought I *had* given my life. I only wanted to be near her, to comfort her. If that's gay, then I was. My feeling as a Christian, in your heart you give up your life for a friend, and love your neighbor as yourself. But I never loved myself before Carol. After I met her, she let me see the 'real' me, the good, loving, and kind person I was. I got a chance to put it into practice. I had finally made it in God's eyes. I, the puzzle piece, finally fit. We think sometimes we are good, and do all that God asks of us, but when we search deep within, we find we really haven't fulfilled His asking. With Carol, I had NO doubt I fulfilled everything He'd asked of me. Finally, true to God, and myself, His Spirit dwelled within me.

Carol changed my life, teaching me love. Loving, I found takes care of all unanswered questions of 'self'. No bad can enter when you are filled with love. I'm glad I met Carol, and honored I was able to care for her and watch her decline. It taught me we are all connected. We all go through decline and finally death, so why is it when it comes our way, we shy away from it? Being with someone who is dying of Alzheimer's, especially because the disease takes so long, watching the decline is a gift. We watch the person 'undo' their life at a slow rate. We may hate watching it, but in the end, I was happy to go through

Carol's Alzheimer's Journey to death. It brought me closer to God than I'd ever been before. Since her body death I know Carol is with me every day. I feel around me: in flowers, trees, flowing waters, skies, birds or insects, like flutterbys to mention a few. She lets me know we are ALL connected.

****

Rose Lamatt

Despair

Sinking deeper into darkness, clawing walls along the way.
Grasping, but not holding, where is the light of day?

Falling faster than the light years, seconds fleeting, one by one.
Heading down so quickly, will the ending never come?

No ending, no beginning, just losing twilight's gleam.
No stars are there appearing, a nightmare or a dream?

Reaching arms out, catch me someone, grab my hands, keep me safe.
Pull me from this downward spiral I am falling throughout space.

Is this the way it feels when your mind is losing pace?
Is this how death will take you? How will you know the place?

As you crawl through tortured chambers, no light comes seeping in.
Do you pay for what you've done in life, for each and every sin?

God send an angel for me, let him lift me with his wings.
Don't let me keep on falling and see what darkness brings.

Will I waken from this endless fall? I need to be touched by someone.
Oh help me, hear my call. Open my eyes quickly, let me see the sun.

And suddenly, the brightness, the pastures and the trees,
the flowers and the music, the soft and gentle breeze.

I have fallen through the darkness through the spiral of despair.
I found the strength I needed, a lovely breath of air.

How wonderful to be here, where ever is this place.
The fear has left me peaceful, I am smiled on, with grace.

So, if all I have just gone through is what dying is about,
then what was all the fear for? God helped this poor soul out.

By Elsie Duggan © August 2007

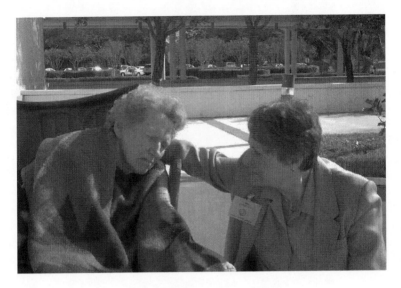

Carol and Rose winter 2004

Rose Lamatt